ABC of

Headache

Anne MacGregor

Director of Clinical Research
The City of London Migraine Clinic

Alison Frith

Clinical Research Sister
The City of London Migraine Clinic

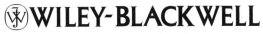
WILEY-BLACKWELL

A John Wiley & Sons, Ltd., Publication

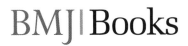
BMJ Books

This edition first published 2009, © 2009 by Blackwell Publishing Ltd

BMJ Books is an imprint of BMJ Publishing Group Limited, used under licence by Blackwell Publishing which was acquired by John Wiley & Sons in February 2007. Blackwell's publishing programme has been merged with Wiley's global Scientific, Technical and Medical business to form Wiley-Blackwell.

Registered office: John Wiley & Sons Ltd, The Atrium, Southern Gate, Chichester, West Sussex, PO19 8SQ, UK

Editorial offices: 9600 Garsington Road, Oxford, OX4 2DQ, UK

The Atrium, Southern Gate, Chichester, West Sussex, PO19 8SQ, UK

111 River Street, Hoboken, NJ 07030-5774, USA

For details of our global editorial offices, for customer services and for information about how to apply for permission to reuse the copyright material in this book please see our website at www.wiley.com/wiley-blackwell

Library of Congress Cataloging-in-Publication Data

ABC of headache / edited by Anne MacGregor, Alison Frith.
     p. ; cm.
   Includes bibliographical references and index.
   ISBN 978-1-4051-7066-6 (alk. paper)
   1. Headache.   I. MacGregor, Anne, 1960–   II. Frith, Alison.
   [DNLM: 1. Headache–diagnosis. 2. Headache Disorders–diagnosis.   WL 342 A112 2008]
   RC392.A27 2008
   616.8′491–dc22

                                    2008001983

ISBN: 978-1-4051-7066-6

A catalogue record for this book is available from the British Library

Set in 9.25/12 pt Minion by SNP Best-set Typesetter Ltd., Hong Kong
Printed in Singapore by COS Printers Pte Ltd

1   2009

Contents

Preface

Our aim with this ABC book is to provide the reader with a clear, concise text to recognize and manage headache effectively. We are grateful for the opportunity to collaborate with colleagues to provide current information based on best available evidence and expert specialist opinion.

First we present an overall approach to headache including eliciting the history, identifying 'red flags' and current issues in investigation and management. The chapters that follow are carefully selected case studies with emphasis on history taking to establish differential diagnoses, investigations that may be required and specific management strategies. Although we illustrate the main primary headaches of migraine, tension-type headache, and cluster headache, we recognize that not all secondary headache types are covered. Obvious headaches due to head trauma or infection for example, have been omitted. Instead, we have chosen common but under-recognized medication overuse headaches and headaches attributed to depression, neck pain and trigeminal neuralgia. Headaches associated with underlying cranial vascular disorder and brain tumours, although rare, are included since they are greatly feared by both patients and health-care professionals.

Individual case studies cannot address all the issues relating to a specific group of headache sufferers. However, we felt it was important to devote chapters on headache and associated syndromes in children and adolescents to highlight their specific issues. With regard to headache in the elderly, the treatments are the same as for other age groups, but the differential diagnosis is particularly important as demonstrated in the chapter on giant cell arteritis. As a quarter of all women are affected by migraine and half of them recognise an association with menstruation, we felt it was appropriate to include a case study for this group.

We hope that this approach to headache reflects presentation of headache to a wide range of healthcare professionals, helping them to improve the diagnosis and the management of this complex and challenging condition.

Anne MacGregor
Alison Frith

Contributors

Ishaq Abu-Arafeh

Consultant Paediatrician
Stirling Royal Infirmary
Stirling, UK

David W. Dodick

Professor of Neurology
Mayo Clinic Arizona
Scottsdale, Arizona, US

Alison Frith

Clinical Research Sister
The City of London Migraine Clinic
London, UK

Anne MacGregor

Director of Clinical Research
The City of London Migraine Clinic
London, UK

R. Allan Purdy

Professor of Medicine (Neurology)
Dalhousie University
Halifax, Nova Scotia, Canada

CHAPTER 1

Approach to Headaches

Anne MacGregor

OVERVIEW

- Most headaches can be managed in primary care
- The history is a crucial step in the correct diagnosis
- Funduscopy is mandatory for anyone presenting with headache
- Diary cards aid diagnosis and management
- The presence of warning symptoms in the history and/or physical signs on examination warrant investigation and may indicate appropriate specialist referral

Introduction

Nearly everyone will experience headaches at some time in their lives. Most headaches are trivial, with an obvious cause and minimal associated disability. However, some headaches are sufficiently troublesome that the person seeks medical help. Headache accounts for 4.4% of consultations in primary care (6.4% females and 2.5% males). Unless a correct diagnosis is made, it is not possible to provide the most effective treatment. For most medical ailments the suspected diagnosis can be confirmed with tests, but no diagnostic test can confirm the most common headaches, such as migraine or tension-type headache. This means that unless the headache is obvious, diagnosis is largely based on the history. In addition, the examination of people with primary headaches is essentially normal. Consequently, the diagnosis is not always easy, particularly if several headaches coexist, confusing both patient and doctor. In a study of patients with a diagnosis of migraine who were referred to a specialist migraine clinic, nearly one third had a headache additional to migraine. Failure to recognize and manage the additional headache was the most common cause of treatment failure.

It is not always possible to confirm the diagnosis at the first visit. A structured history, followed by a relevant examination, can identify patients who need immediate investigations or referral from the non-urgent cases. Management and follow-up will depend on whether the diagnosis is confidently ascertained or is uncertain (Figure 1.1).

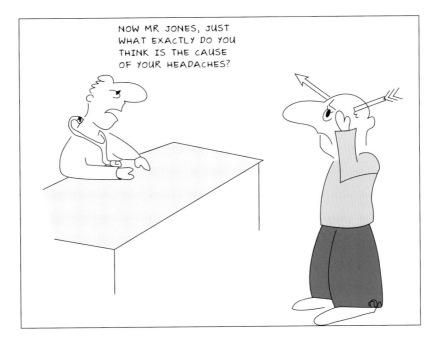

ABC of Headache. Edited by A. MacGregor & A. Frith.
© 2009 Blackwell Publishing, ISBN 978-1-4051-7066-6.

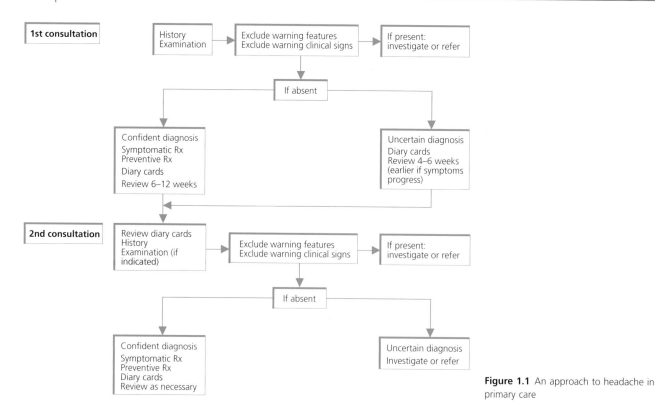

Figure 1.1 An approach to headache in primary care

Table 1.1 An approach to the headache history

1. *How many different headache types does the patient experience?*	

Separate histories are necessary for each. It is reasonable to concentrate on the most bothersome to the patient but others should always attract some enquiry in case they are clinically important.

2. *Time questions*	a)	Why consulting now?
	b)	How recent in onset?
	c)	How frequent and what temporal pattern (especially distinguishing between episodic and daily or unremitting)?
	d)	How long lasting?
3. *Character questions*	a)	Intensity of pain?
	b)	Nature and quality of pain?
	c)	Site and spread of pain?
	d)	Associated symptoms?
4. *Cause questions*	a)	Predisposing and/or trigger factors?
	b)	Aggravating and/or relieving factors?
	c)	Family history of similar headache?
5. *Response to headache questions*	a)	What does the patient do during the headache?
	b)	How much is activity (function) limited or prevented?
	c)	What medication has been and is used, and in what manner?
6. *State of health between attacks*	a)	Completely well, or residual or persisting symptoms?
	b)	Concerns, anxieties, fears about recurrent attacks and/or their cause?

Source: Steiner TJ, MacGregor EA, Davies PTG. *Guidelines for All Healthcare Professionals in the Diagnosis and Management of Migraine, Tension-Type, Cluster and Medication Overuse Headache* (3rd edition, 2007). www.bash.org.uk

History

The history is a crucial step in diagnosis of headaches (Table 1.1). A separate history is required for each type of headache reported, in particular noting the course and duration of each. The International Headache Society has developed classification and diagnostic criteria for the majority of primary and secondary headaches (Box 1.1). Although this is primarily a research tool, standardized diagnostic criteria have helped to ascertain headache prevalence, which is useful for understanding the likelihood of any headache presenting in clinical practice (Tables 1.2 and 1.3).

A headache history requires time. In the emergency setting particularly, there may not be enough time to take a full history. The first task is to exclude a condition requiring more urgent intervention by identifying any warning features in the history (Box 1.2).

Box 1.1 *The International Classification of Headache Disorders* (2nd edition)

Primary headache

1. Migraine, including:
   - Migraine without aura
   - Migraine with aura
   - Childhood periodic syndromes that are commonly precursors of migraine
   - Cyclical vomiting
   - Abdominal migraine
   - Benign paroxysmal vertigo of childhood
2. Tension-type headache, including:
   - Infrequent episodic tension-type headache
   - Frequent episodic tension-type headache
   - Chronic tension-type headache
3. Cluster headache and other trigeminal autonomic cephalalgias, including:
   - Cluster headache
   - Paroxysmal hemicrania
   - Short-lasting unilateral neuralgiform headache attacks with conjunctival injection and tearing
4. Other primary headaches, including:
   - Primary cough headache
   - Primary exertional headache
   - Primary headache associated with sexual activity
   - Primary thunderclap headache

Secondary headache

5. Headache attributed to head and/or neck trauma, including:
   - Chronic post-traumatic headache
6. Headache attributed to cranial or cervical vascular disorder, including:
   - Headache attributed to subarachnoid haemorrhage
   - Headache attributed to giant cell arteritis
7. Headache attributed to non-vascular intracranial disorder, including:
   - Headache attributed to idiopathic intracranial hypertension
   - Headache attributed to low cerebrospinal fluid pressure
   - Headache attributed to non-infectious inflammatory disease
   - Headache attributed to intracranial neoplasm
8. Headache attributed to a substance or its withdrawal, including:
   - Carbon monoxide-induced headache
   - Alcohol-induced headache
   - Medication-overuse headache
   - Triptan-overuse headache
   - Analgesic-overuse headache
9. Headache attributed to infection, including:
   - Headache attributed to intracranial infection
10. Headache attributed to disorder of homoeostasis
11. Headache or facial pain attributed to disorder of cranium, neck, eyes, ears, nose, sinuses, teeth, mouth or other facial or cranial structures, including:
    - Cervicogenic headache
    - Headache attributed to acute glaucoma
12. Headache attributed to psychiatric disorder

Neuralgias and other headaches

13. Cranial neuralgias and central causes of facial pain including:
    - Trigeminal neuralgia
14. Other headache, cranial neuralgia, central or primary facial pain

Appendix (unvalidated research criteria)

Including:
- Pure menstrual migraine without aura
- Menstrually-related migraine without aura
- Benign paroxysmal torticollis
- Headache attributed to major depressive disorder

Source: adapted from Headache Classification Subcommittee of the International Headache Society (IHS). *The International Classification of Headache Disorders* (2nd edition). *Cephalalgia* 2004; **24** (suppl 1): 1–160.

New or recently changed headache calls for especially careful assessment. New headache in any patient over 50 years of age should raise the suspicion of giant cell arteritis (Chapter 14). Headache is likely to be persistent when present, often worse at night and may be very severe. Jaw claudication is so suggestive that its presence confirms the diagnosis until proved otherwise. In the absence of 'red flags', strictly unilateral headaches may suggest a common headache, such as migraine (Chapter 2) or one of the more rare trigeminal autonomic cephalalgias (Chapter 4).

An uncommon but avoidable cause of non-specific headache in elderly patients is carbon monoxide poisoning. This is caused by using gas heaters, which may be faulty, without adequate ventila-tion. The symptoms of sub-acute carbon monoxide poisoning include throbbing headache, nausea, vomiting, giddiness and fatigue.

The major fear among patients and healthcare professionals is that a brain tumour is the cause of the headache. In practice, intracranial lesions (tumours, subarachnoid haemorrhage, menin-gitis) give rise to histories that should bring them to mind. It is rare for brain tumours and other serious conditions to present as isolated headache (Table 1.4). Epilepsy is a cardinal symptom of intracerebral space-occupying lesions, and loss of consciousness should be viewed very seriously. Problems are more likely to occur with slow-growing tumours, especially those in neurologically 'silent' areas of the frontal lobes. Subtle personality change may result in treatment for depression, with headache attributed to it. Heightened suspicion is appropriate in patients who develop new

Table 1.2 Lifetime prevalence of primary headaches

Type of headache	Prevalence % (95% CI)
Migraine without aura	9 (7–11)
Migraine with aura	6 (5–8)
Episodic tension-type headache	66 (62–69)
Chronic tension-type headache	3 (2–5)
Cluster headache	0.1 (0–1)

Source: Rasmussen BK. Epidemiology of headache. *Cephalalgia* 1995; **15**: 45–68.

Table 1.3 Lifetime prevalence of secondary headaches

Type of headache	Prevalence % (95% CI)
Head trauma	4 (2–5)
Vascular disorders	1 (0–2)
Non-vascular cranial disorders	0.5 (0–1)
Substances or their withdrawal (excluding hangover)	3 (2–4)
– hangover	72 (68–75)
Non-cephalic infection	63 (59–66)
Metabolic disorder	22 (19–25)
Disorders of the cranium, neck, eyes	0.5–3 (0–4)
– sinuses	15 (12–17)
Cranial neuralgias	0.5 (0–1)

Source: Rasmussen BK. Epidemiology of headache, *Cephalalgia* 1995; **15**: 45–68.

Box 1.2 **Warning features in the history warranting investigation**

- Acute thunderclap headache (intense headache with abrupt or 'explosive' onset)
- Headache with atypical aura (duration >1 hour, or including motor weakness)
- New onset headache in a patient younger than 10 years or older than 50 years
- Progressive headache, worsening over weeks or longer
- Fever
- Symptoms of raised intracranial pressure:
    drowsiness
    postural-related headache
    vomiting
- New onset seizures
- History of cancer or HIV infection
- Cognitive or personality changes
- Progressive neurological deficit:
    progressive weakness
    sensory loss
    dysphasia
    ataxia

Table 1.4 Secondary causes of headache identified in the year after presentation in primary care of a primary headache or new undifferentiated headache

Subsequent secondary diagnosis	Headache diagnosis at presentation n (%)	
	New undifferentiated headache n = 63 921	Primary headache n = 21 758
Subarachnoid haemorrhage	87 (0.14)	5 (0.02)
Malignant brain tumour	97 (0.15)	10 (0.045)
Benign space-occupying lesion	30 (0.05)	2 (0.009)
Temporal arteritis	421 (0.66)	40 (0.18)
Stroke	678 (1.06)	97 (0.45)
Transient ischaemic attack	273 (0.43)	54 (0.25)

Source: Based on Kernick D et al. What happens to new onset headache presented to primary care? A case-cohort study using electronic primary care records. *Cephalalgia* (2008 forthcoming).

headache and are known to have cancer elsewhere or a suppressed immune system.

Examination

In primary care time is of the essence, not just to make the diagnosis, but to do so in such a way that the patient can be reassured. A recent outpatient study found only 0.9% of consecutive headache patients without neurological signs had significant pathology. This reinforces the importance of physical examination in diagnosing serious causes of headache.

The examination must be thorough but can be brief. A quick neurological examination for recurrent headache has been devised to elicit the most likely pathological findings, if present (Table 1.5). If any clinical signs are present, a more detailed examination is indicated.

Table 1.5 The neurological examination

While patient is standing

Ask the patient to:	Tests:
Close your eyes and stand with your feet together (Romberg)	Midline cerebellar; dorsal column; proprioception
Open your eyes and walk heel to toe	Midline cerebellar; dorsal column; proprioception
Walk on your tiptoes	Power of dorsiflexion
Walk on your heels	Power of plantar flexion
Close your eyes and hold your hands out straight in front of you with your palms flat and facing upwards	Hemisphere lesions (e.g. left hemisphere lesion, right hand will bend in and drift up) Neglect (e.g. left parietal lesion, right hand will drop down)
Keep your eyes closed. Touch your nose with the fingertip that I touch (person testing uses their own finger to touch a couple of the patient's fingertips in turn)	Light touch and finger–nose test (cerebellar or sensory ataxia and light-touch in fingertip)
Open your eyes and with your arms outstretched, pretend to play the piano	Fine finger movements Pyramidal and extrapyramidal function
Tap the back of one hand with your other hand. Change hands and repeat	Ataxia
Screw your eyes up tight and then relax and open your eyes	Pupil dilation and constriction Horner's syndrome Lower motor neurone lesion
Bare your teeth/grin	Upper motor neurone facial weakness
Stick your tongue out and wiggle it	Bulbar and pseudobulbar palsy
Stare at my face and point at the fingers which move (person testing has arms out to the side with index finger pointing. Arms stop in an arc and index finger is wiggled on each side in turn or together)	Temporal field defects (important visual field defects always involve one or other temporal field) Inattention (parietal lobe lesion)
Keeping your head still, stare at my finger and follow it up and down with your eyes (person testing draws a wide 'H' in the air)	Eye movements (cranial nerves III, IV, VI) Nystagmus; saccadic (jerky) eye movements

While patient is lying down

Examine:	Tests:
Limb reflexes	Upper motor neurone lesion (brisk) Peripheral nerve or nerve root lesion (absent)
Plantar response	Upper motor neurone lesion (Babinski/extensor response)
Abdominal reflexes	Spinal cord disease
Funduscopy	Raised intracranial pressure (papilloedema) Optic atrophy
Pulse and blood pressure	Hypertension
If indicated, examine the chest, palpate breasts and abdomen	Systemic disease, e.g. neoplasia

Source: based on Elrington G. How to do a neurological examination in five minutes or less. *Pulse*, 2 October 2007: www.pulsetoday.co.uk

If there is insufficient time even for such a brief examination, it can be deferred to a later date provided that the optic fundi have been examined. Funduscopic examination is mandatory at first presentation with headache, and it is always worthwhile to repeat it during follow-up.

Blood pressure measurement is recommended: raised blood pressure is very rarely a cause of headache, but patients often think it may be. Raised blood pressure may make headache of other causes, including migraine, more difficult to treat unless it is itself treated. Drugs used for headache, especially migraine and cluster headache, affect blood pressure, and vice versa.

Examine the head and neck for muscle tenderness (generalized or with tender 'nodules'), stiffness, limitation in range of movement and crepitation. Positive findings may suggest a need for physical forms of treatment but not necessarily headache causation. It is uncertain whether routine examination of the jaw and bite contribute to headache diagnosis, but it may reveal incidental abnormalities.

In children, some paediatricians recommend that head circumference is measured at the diagnostic visit and plotted on a centile chart. Weight is important when considering the dose of medication and, together with height, can indicate normal growth.

Investigations

In clinical practice, the initial concern is differentiation of primary headaches from secondary, sinister headaches.

Investigations, including neuroimaging, do not contribute to the diagnosis of primary headaches and are not warranted in children or adults with a defined headache and normal neurological examination. They are necessary only if secondary headache is suspected because of undefined headache, atypical symptoms, persistent neurological or psychopathological abnormalities, abnormal findings on neurological examination or recent trauma. A low threshold is indicated for new onset headaches and if there is significant parental anxiety about a child with headache. Inappropriate investigations can increase morbidity, particularly in the presence of unrelated incidental findings and, with respect to computed tomography, unnecessary radiation exposure.

- *Full blood count and erythrocyte sedimentation rate* may detect the presence of infection or giant cell arteritis.
- *Plain radiography* of the skull is normal in most patients with headache, but may be indicated if there is a history of head injury or if symptoms/examination are suggestive of a tumour, particularly of the pituitary gland. Cervical spine x-rays are usually unhelpful, even when neck signs suggest origin from the neck, as they do not alter management.
- *Lumbar puncture* confirms infection (e.g. meningitis or encephalitis). It should be used if subarachnoid haemorrhage is suspected (e.g. acute thunderclap headache) and CT is either unavailable or the results are inconclusive – CT may be normal in 10–15% of all subarachnoid haemorrhage.
- *Electro-encephalography (EEG)* is of little diagnostic value in migraine but may be considered if a clinical diagnosis suggests features of epilepsy, such as loss of consciousness occurring in association with migraine.

- *Computed tomography (CT)* demonstrates structural lesions, including tumour, vascular malformations, haemorrhage and hydrocephalus. If intracranial or subarachnoid haemorrhage is suspected, CT scan without contrast can detect recent bleeds; MRI may miss fresh blood. It may be necessary to give an intravenous injection of contrast material to highlight a suspected tumour or vascular lesion. Indications for CT are persistent focal neurological deficits, symptoms or signs suggestive of an arteriovenous malformation and haemorrhagic stroke.
- *Magnetic resonance imaging (MRI)* produces better definition of soft tissue abnormalities than CT scanning and is the investigation of choice for cerebral infarction. MRI with gadolinium is the investigation of choice for meningeal pathology. Although CT can detect most tumours, MRI is more sensitive as it can detect both infiltrating and very small tumours.
- *Cerebral angiography* is rarely required as a primary investigation and its use is limited by its invasiveness. If CT or MRI confirms arteriovenous malformation, angiography is used to define the extent of the lesion and demonstrate feeding and draining vessels.
- *Isotope scanning* and *Doppler flow studies* are mostly only of value for research.

Headache diaries

Patients should be asked to keep a daily record of all their symptoms and all treatments taken for headache, including dose and time(s) taken. The pattern of attacks is a very helpful pointer to the right diagnosis, particularly if the diagnosis is unclear or more than one type of headache is present. If the patient has migraine, a clear pattern of episodic headaches will be apparent, with freedom from symptoms between attacks (Figure 1.2). Failure to respond to standard treatment strategies for the considered diagnosis is an alert for close review. More often than not, several headaches coexist and each needs to be considered separately. Diary cards can help distinguish the different headache types. For example, migraine attacks may be evident as more severe headache with nausea on a background of daily headache (Figure 1.3). Medication overuse should always be excluded in anyone using symptomatic treatments for headache more often than 2–3 days a week.

Review of diary cards can also identify what medication is taken and if it is taken in adequate doses at the optimal time.

Managing the undiagnosed headache

In a study of patients presenting to UK primary care with new onset headache, 24% were diagnosed with a primary headache disorder (73% migraine, 23% tension-type, 4% cluster) and 6% were diagnosed with a secondary headache, of which 83% were coded as 'sinus' headache.

Once a diagnosis of primary headache has been made, the risk of the headache being consequent to a secondary cause is low (Table 1.4). However, 70% of headaches in the UK primary care study were not given a diagnosis. In these cases, watchful waiting for the development of additional signs or symptoms, with regular monitoring (particularly in the young and old) is recommended.

Month. June.......... Year. 2007.......... Other Drugs: Daily Preventative: Name. None....... Dose.................
Name. A.N Other. DOB. 15/04/1960..   Hormonal Treatments: Name. None.................................

Date	Day	Headache or Migraine	Severity	Time Started	Nausea	Vomiting	What treatment did you take	Time taken
1	MON							
2	TUE							
3	WED	migraine	Severe	4 am	Yes	Yes	Triptan	4 am & 1 pm
4	THU							
5	FRI							
6	SAT							
7	SUN							
8	MON							
9	TUE							
10	WED							
11	THU	headache	mild	7 pm	No	No	Analgesic	9.30 pm
12	FRI	headache	moderate	10 am	Yes	No	Analgesic	10 pm
13	SAT							
14	SUN							
15	MON							

Figure 1.2 Headache diary: episodic headaches

Month. June.......... Year. 2007.......... Other Drugs: Daily Preventative: Name. None....... Dose.................
Name. O.V.Dose. DOB. 11/11/1950..   Hormonal Treatments: Name. None.................................

Date	Day	Headache or Migraine	Severity	Time Started	Nausea	Vomiting	What treatment did you take	Time taken
1	MON	H	mod	5.10 am	no	no	analgesic	5.10 am
2	TUE	H	mod	5.00 am	no	no	analgesic	5.00 am
3	WED	H	mod	5.00 am	no	no	analgesic	5.00 am
4	THU	H	mod	5.30 am	no	no	analgesic	5.30 am
5	FRI	migraine	severe	6.00 am	Yes	no	triptan	6.00 am
6	SAT	H	mod	6.10 am	Yes	no	triptan	6.10 am
7	SUN	–	–	–	–	–	–	–
8	MON	migraine	severe	4.30 am	Yes	Yes	triptan	7 am/3 pm
9	TUE	migraine	severe	4.30 am	Yes	no	triptan	4.30 am
10	WED	migraine	severe	3.00 am	Yes	no	triptan	3 am/7 am
11	THU	H	mod	7.00 am	no	no	analgesic	7.00 am
12	FRI	H	mod	12.10 am	no	no	analgesic	12.10 am
13	SAT	H	mod	7.00 am	no	no	analgesic	7.00 am
14	SUN	H	mod	7.30 am	no	no	analgesic	7.30 am
15	MON	H	mod	7.10 am	no	no	analgesic	7.10 am

Figure 1.3 Headache diary: daily headaches (possible medication overuse) with migraine

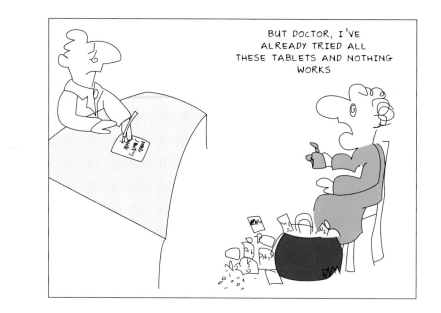

In most cases, a pattern emerges within 3–6 months, resulting in the majority of cases being given a correct diagnosis.

Further reading

Blau JN, MacGregor EA. Migraine consultations: a triangle of viewpoints. *Headache* 1995; **35(2)**: 104–6.

Elrington G. How to do a neurological examination in five minutes or less. *Pulse*, 2 October 2007: www.pulsetoday.co.uk

Kernick D, Stapley S, Hamilton W. What happens to new onset headache presented to primary care? A case-cohort study using electronic primary care records. *Cephalalgia* (2008 forthcoming).

Latinovic R, Gulliford M, Ridsdale L. Headache and migraine in primary care: consultation, prescription, and referral rates in a large population. *J Neurol Neurosurg Psychiatry* 2006; **77(3)**: 385–7.

Steiner TJ, MacGregor EA, Davies PTG. *Guidelines for All Healthcare Professionals in the Diagnosis and Management of Migraine, Tension-Type, Cluster and Medication Overuse Headache* (3rd edition, 2007). www.bash.org.uk

Stovner L, Hagen K, Jensen R, et al. The global burden of headache: a documentation of headache prevalence and disability worldwide. *Cephalalgia* 2007; **27(3)**: 193–210.

CHAPTER 2

Migraine

Anne MacGregor

OVERVIEW

- Recurrent, episodic 'sick' headaches in an otherwise well person are likely to be migraine
- The history is important as on examination there are no clinical signs
- Diary cards can aid diagnosis and assessment of response to treatment
- Referral is indicated if the diagnosis is unclear or there is no response to standard treatment strategies

CASE HISTORY

The man with episodic sick headaches

KH is 37. He presents with severe headache associated with nausea. The headache is typically present on waking and worsens over the course of the morning. The pain starts in the temples, affecting the right more than the left side and is temporarily eased by pressure. From the temples, the pain gradually spreads to settle in the back of the head. He always feels nauseous, but only vomits occasionally during particularly severe attacks. Eventually he has to stop what he is doing and lie down in a darkened room.

Occasionally, KH gets a warning before the attack starts, with a bright spot in his vision, which slowly expands over about 20 minutes before disappearing. It is followed by headache.

History

How many different headache types does the patient experience?

KH responds that he has one type of headache. Although he has visual symptoms before some attacks, the headache is the same but less severe.

Time questions

KH is losing time from work, which is a problem. His first attack was when he was 11 when he suddenly noticed bright zigzag lines in front of his eyes. He had a severe headache with vomiting which resolved after a few hours. Now attacks are every 10–14 days. They used to be at weekends but since he has started doing shift work, they can come at any time. Attacks can last up to three days.

Character questions

The intensity varies from a dull nagging ache to a severe throbbing headache. It usually starts in the right temple, spreads across to the left side and down into the back of the neck. It is tender to touch. KH feels sick and does not want to eat, although he only vomits occasionally. He retires to a quiet, dark room as light and sound bother him.

Cause questions

KH used to get attacks more often after a busy week at work or the first couple of days of a holiday. Sleep and keeping still with a cool pad over his eyes both help. He finds it difficult to sleep because of the pain. His grandmother used to get 'sick' headaches.

Response to headache questions

KH has to stop his usual activities and lie down. Over the last month, he has been absent from work for two days because of the attacks. Paracetamol used to give some relief but has become less effective. He has tried other over-the-counter painkillers, with limited success.

State of health between attacks

KH reports that he is 'fine' apart from the headaches. He does not think he has 'a brain tumour or anything' since he has had the headaches for so long. However, he is concerned that they are interfering with his life and he is unable to control them.

Examination

Blood pressure 120/75. Funduscopy and brief neurological examination were unremarkable.

Investigations

As there are no sinister symptoms in the history and no abnormal findings on physical examination, there is no indication for investigations.

ABC of Headache. Edited by A. MacGregor & A. Frith.
© 2009 Blackwell Publishing, ISBN 978-1-4051-7066-6.

Diagnosis

Differential diagnosis

In the absence of clinical signs, a primary headache is likely (Figure 2.1). Sinusitis is often mistaken for migraine, although the typical features of discoloured mucus and history of a cold are absent. The main differential diagnosis of aura is transient ischaemic attack (Table 2.1). Migraine auras usually follow a similar pattern for each

attack, although the duration of aura may vary. Therefore, a long history of similar attacks, particularly if onset is in childhood or early adult life, is reassuring. If aura symptoms suddenly change, further investigation may be warranted.

Preliminary diagnosis

Migraine is the probable diagnosis for recurrent, episodic 'sick' headaches in an otherwise well person. A review of four studies of

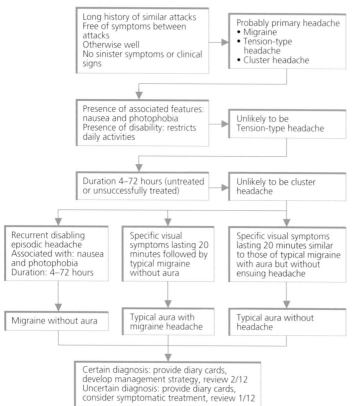

Figure 2.1 Flowchart of differential diagnosis of primary headache

Table 2.1 Distinguishing migraine aura from a transient ischaemic attack

	Migraine	Transient ischaemic attack
History	First attack usually in teens/20s	First attack usually in older population
Onset and progression of symptoms	Slow evolution over several minutes	Sudden (seconds)
Duration	<1 hour (typically 20–30 mins)	Variable – 2 minutes–24 hours
Timing	Precedes and resolves before onset of typical migraine headache	Occurs with or without headache, with no temporal relationship
Visual symptoms	Present in 99% of auras Homonymous positive (bright) scotoma gradually enlarging across visual field into a scintillating crescent	Monocular, negative (black) scotoma (amaurosis fugax)
Sensory/motor symptoms	Present in one-third of auras – usually in association with visual symptoms Rarely affects legs Positive ('pins and needles')	May occur without visual symptoms May include legs Negative (loss of power)
Headache	Aura resolves before onset of headache and associated symptoms	Up to 25% associated with concurrent headache

screening questions for migraine in patients with headache identified five predictors: pulsating, duration 4–72 hours, unilateral, nausea and disabling. If three predictors are present, the likelihood ratio for migraine is 3.5 (95%CI, 1.3–9.2), increasing to 24 (95%CI, 1.5–388) if four predictors are present.

Migraine without aura is a recurrent, episodic, moderate or severe headache lasting part of a day or up to three days, associated with gastrointestinal symptoms and a preference for dark and quiet (Box 2.1). Usual activities are limited in more than three-quarters of sufferers, with one-third needing to lie down. Between attacks, people with typical migraine are free of symptoms and are otherwise well.

Migraine with aura describes a complex of neurological symptoms that usually progress over 5–60 minutes and resolve completely before the onset of headache (Box 2.2). Attacks with aura are more prevalent with increasing age and the headache may be mild or completely absent. Visual symptoms are common, experienced in 99% of auras. The typical 'fortification spectra' begins with a small bright scotoma that gradually increases in size, developing zigzag scintillating edges (Figure 2.2). When asked to describe the symptoms patients may draw a jagged crescent. Visual symptoms occur together or in sequence, with other reversible focal neurological disturbances such as dysphasia and/or a tingling sensation of 'pins and needles' spreading from the hand into the face. The leg is rarely affected. Transient monocular blindness, atypical or prolonged aura, especially aura persisting after resolution of the headache, and aura involving motor weakness require referral for exclusion of other disease.

Initial management

This includes:
- reassurance
- symptomatic treatment

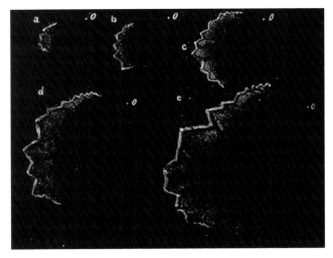

Figure 2.2 Progression of symptoms of migraine visual aura
Source: Airy H. On a distinct form of transient hemiopsia. *Phil Trans Roy Soc* 1870; **160**: 247–64.

Table 2.2 Common predisposing and triggering factors for migraine

Factor	Management summary
Stress	Lifestyle change; stress reduction/coping strategies
Dehydration	Drink minimum 1.5 L fluids per day
Depression/anxiety	Specific therapy
Menstruation	See chapter 6
Head or neck trauma	Physiotherapy
Relaxation after stress, especially at weekends or on holiday	Stress avoidance; lifestyle change
Other change in habit: missing meals; missing sleep; lying in late; long-distance travel	Avoidance if possible; otherwise avoidance of additional triggers
Bright lights and loud noise (both perhaps stress-inducing)	Avoidance
Dietary: certain alcoholic drinks; some cheeses	Avoidance if indicated
Strenuous, unaccustomed exercise	Keeping fit /avoidance

Date	Day	Headache or Migraine	Severity	Time Started	Did you feel sick	Were you sick	What tablets did you take	What time taken
1	TUE							
2	WED							
3	THU							
4	FRI							
5	SAT							
6	SUN							
7	MON							
8	TUE	Migraine	MOD	1 am	Yes	No	Triptan	1 pm
9	WED	Migraine	SEV	8 am	Yes	No	Triptan	8 am
10	THU							
11	FRI	Headache	MILD	9 am	No	No	Analgesic	7 am
12	SAT							
13	SUN							
14	MON							

Figure 2.3 Example of a diary card

- discussion of potential predisposing and triggering factors (Table 2.2)
- diary cards to confirm diagnosis, assess frequency and duration of attacks, and response to symptomatic treatment (Figure 2.3)
- review after 4–8 weeks

Symptomatic treatment

Symptomatic drugs are the mainstay of management but should be restricted to no more than three days a week (10–15 days a month) to prevent medication overuse headache.

Analgesics and anti-emetics

Initial treatment with an analgesic, often combined with a prokinetic anti-emetic, is a reasonable choice for mild to moderate migraine (Tables 2.3–2.5). In addition to reversing the gastric stasis that accompanies migraine, gastroprokinetic agents may have the advantage of enhancing the bioavailability of concomitant drugs given orally.

Chlorpromazine (25–50 mg im), metoclopramide (10 mg iv or im) and prochlorperazine (10 mg iv or im) have also been used as single-agent therapies in migraine with success and should be considered for emergency treatment of migraine.

Table 2.3 Simple analgesics

Analgesic	Initial dose	Dose frequency	Max. daily
Aspirin	900 mg	Repeat second dose at two hours, thereafter four-hourly	4 g
Paracetamol	1000 mg	Every 4–6 hours	4 g
Ibuprofen	600–800 mg	Every 4–6 hours	2.4 g

Table 2.4 Non-steroidal anti-inflammatory drugs

Drug	Initial dose	Dose frequency	Max. daily
Diclofenac	Oral or rectal: 100 mg	50–100 mg after six hours	200 mg
Naproxen	Oral: 750 mg	250 mg after 4–6 hours	1250 mg
Tolfenamic acid	Oral: 200 mg	200 mg after 2–3 hours	400 mg

Table 2.5 Prokinetic anti-emetics

Anti-emetic	Initial dose	Dose frequency	Max. daily
Domperidone	Oral: 20–30 mg	Every 4–6 hours	80 mg
	Rectal: 30–60 mg	Every 4–8 hours	120 mg
Metoclopramide	Oral: 10 mg	Every 6–8 hours	30 mg

Table 2.6 Triptans

Use	Dose regimen
Appropriate for first use of a triptan	Almotriptan 12.5 mg, eletriptan 40 mg, sumatriptan 50 mg or zolmitriptan 2.5 mg oral
When greater efficacy is needed	Eletriptan 80 mg or rizatriptan 10 mg, sumatriptan 100 mg or zolmitriptan 5 mg oral, or sumatriptan 20 mg intranasal
When a rapid response is important above all	Sumatriptan 6 mg subcutaneous or zolmitriptan 5 mg intranasal
When nausea or vomiting precludes oral therapy	Sumatriptan 6 mg subcutaneous or zolmitriptan 5 mg intranasal
When side-effects are troublesome with other triptans	Naratriptan 2.5 mg or almotriptan 12.5 mg or frovatriptan 2.5 mg oral

Source: adapted from Steiner TJ, MacGregor EA, Davies PTG. *Guidelines for All Healthcare Professionals in the Diagnosis and Management of Migraine, Tension-Type, Cluster and Medication Overuse Headache* (3rd edition 2007). www.bash.org.uk

Triptans

Seven triptans are available (Table 2.6). Triptans are likely to be ineffective if taken during aura and should be taken at onset of headache. If migraine relapses after successful treatment, a second dose of triptan can be given. A triptan combined with a non-steroidal anti-inflammatory drug (NSAID) may reduce the likelihood of relapse.

Table 2.7 Ergotamine

Route	Dose	Max. doses/week
Oral	1–2 mg	2
Rectal	1–2 mg (1/2–1 suppository)	2

Ergot derivatives

Ergot derivatives may be considered if recurrent relapse with triptans is a significant problem (Table 2.7). Toxicity and misuse potential are greater than with triptans, so the frequency of intake should be restricted to a maximum of 10 days a month.

Referral

Since the diagnosis is unlikely to be other than migraine, there is no indication to refer KH unless his symptoms fail to respond to standard management strategies.

Management plan

KH opts to try an analgesic and anti-emetic at the onset of symptoms. He is also prescribed a triptan to take if this strategy is insufficient. He is advised that if he consistently requires a triptan, he should use this as first-line treatment. He will keep a diary of attacks and is keen to identify potential triggers.

Final diagnosis

Eight weeks later, review of KH's diary cards shows episodic headache with complete freedom from symptoms between attacks, confirming the diagnosis of migraine with and without aura.

Ongoing management

Although the response to symptomatic treatment has been good, KH has still lost time from work. Whilst he thinks that lack of food and dehydration are significant factors, he is keen to try other strategies.

Prophylactic drugs aim to reduce the frequency, duration and severity of migraine attacks (Box 2.3). Overall, about one-third of patients who are treated with prophylactic agents can be expected to have a 50% reduction in the frequency of their headaches.

Prophylactic treatment
Beta-blockers

Atenolol* 25–100 mg bd, metoprolol 50–100 mg bd or propranolol 20–80 mg bd are first-line options.

Antidepressants

Amitriptyline* 10–150 mg daily, taken 1–2 hours before bedtime, is first-line treatment when migraine coexists with troublesome

---

* Unlicensed indication.

Box 2.3 **Prophylactic management of migraine**

- Confirm that the patient wishes to take prophylaxis
- Discuss expectations and ensure that the patient understands that complete suppression of migraine is unlikely
- Start with medications that have the highest level of evidence-based efficacy
- Start with the lowest dose and increase it slowly until clinical benefits are achieved for the patient in the absence of, or until limited by, adverse effects
- Give each medication an adequate trial as it can take 2–3 months to achieve benefit in some cases
- Consider reducing the dose or even discontinuing the medication if, after 3–6 months, headaches are well controlled
- Single daily doses may improve compliance compared to multiple daily doses
- Establish that any agent chosen is not contraindicated in any coexisting illness or pregnancy plans
- Choose an agent that may be beneficial in any coexisting illness

tension-type headache, another chronic pain condition, disturbed sleep or depression. Low doses should be used initially, increasing by 10 mg every two weeks until symptoms are controlled.

Anti-epileptic drugs/neuromodulators

Topiramate 25–50 mg bd and sodium valproate* 300–1000 mg bd are second-line options. Evidence for the use of other antiepileptics, such as gabapentin and lamotrigine, is weak.

Calcium-channel blockers

The evidence is best for the use of flunarizine, which has equivalent efficacy to propranolol and metoprolol. It is a second-line agent because side-effects, including weight gain, are more apparent than with first-line agents. Trials for the use of other calcium channel blockers have given mixed results.

Serotonin antagonists

Methysergide 1–2 mg tds is generally considered the most effective prophylactic, but is held in reserve as a third-line agent. This is partly because of its association with retroperitoneal fibrosis, although this is unlikely to occur in courses of less than six months.

There are few data to support the use of pizotifen, and sedation and weight gain are common.

Alternative prophylaxis

Limited data from randomized placebo-controlled trials suggest that the following may reduce attack frequency and are well tolerated:

- Riboflavin (vitamin B2) 400 mg daily (more than 20 times the recommended daily intake)
- Coenzyme Q10 (CoQ10) 3×100 mg daily
- Butterbur (*Petasites hybridus*) 75 mg daily

There are limited data for feverfew and no good data on transcutaneous electrical nerve stimulation (TENS), occlusal adjustment, cervical manipulation or physiotherapy. Sham acupuncture is as effective as acupuncture.

Relaxation training, biofeedback and cognitive behavioural therapy show some effect in preventing migraine.

Outcome

Symptomatic treatment with an NSAID, together with a prokinetic anti-emetic, was not as effective as a triptan for KH, but the latter was associated with relapse of symptoms over a couple of days. Beta-blockers reduced the frequency and severity of attacks, which were less likely to relapse when treated with a triptan. KH considered lifestyle triggers and after three months of treatment was able to stop prophylaxis and maintain control with symptomatic treatment only.

Further reading

Detsky ME, McDonald DR, Baerlocker MO, Tomlinson GA, McCory DC, Booth CM. Does this patient with headache have a migraine or need neuroimaging? *JAMA* 2006; **296**: 1274–83.

Ferrari MD, Goadsby PJ, Roon KI, Lipton RB. Triptans (serotonin, 5-HT1B/1D agonists) in migraine: detailed results and methods of a meta-analysis of 53 trials. *Cephalalgia* 2002; **22(8)**: 633–58.

Lipton RB, Dodick D, Sadovsky R, et al. A self-administered screener for migraine in primary care: The ID migraine validation study. *Neurology* 2003; **61(3)**: 375–82.

Silberstein SD. Migraine. *Lancet* 2004; **363(9406)**: 381–91.

Steiner TJ, MacGregor EA, Davies PTG. *Guidelines for All Healthcare Professionals in the Diagnosis and Management of Migraine, Tension-Type, Cluster and Medication Overuse Headache* (3rd edition 2007): www.bash.org.uk

* Unlicensed indication.

CHAPTER 3

Tension-type Headache

Anne MacGregor

OVERVIEW

- Headaches that lack associated symptoms in an otherwise well person who is not overusing medication are likely to be tension-type headaches
- The history is important as on examination there are no significant clinical signs, although pericranial muscle tenderness may be present
- Diary cards can aid diagnosis and assessment of response to treatment
- Referral is indicated if the diagnosis is unclear or there is no response to standard treatment strategies

CASE HISTORY

The woman with 'daily' headaches
EL is a 27-year-old mini-cab driver and does shift work. She presents with troublesome headaches, which she gets most days. The headache can come on at any time of the day. Sometimes the pain is on the left side of her head, but more often it is like a band across the back of her head. There are no associated symptoms. The headaches do not stop her working, but they affect her ability to concentrate.

History

How many different headache types does the patient experience?

EL responds that she has two types of headache. She has had 'sick' headaches since her teens, which she still gets once or twice a year. She recognizes these as migraine. As she knows what they are and can cope with them, they do not concern her. She has come because of daily headaches, which are very different from her migraines.

Time questions

Her more recent headache started a couple of years ago, not long after she started her driving job. She noticed that by the end of a shift she had a headache across the back of her head. Over the last six months or so, she has the headache almost continuously.

Character questions

EL describes the pain as a tightening feeling across the back and sides of her head. It can be painful to touch. There are no other associated symptoms.

Cause questions

EL feels that her job has something to do with the headaches as she did not have them before. She does not cope well with shift work and takes a lot less physical exercise than she used to. The headache is not affected by routine physical activity. She is under financial pressure to take on as much work as she can, and for the last few months has worked most days.

Response to headache questions

EL can continue her daily activities, but the headaches affect her concentration. She has not lost any time from work. She takes ibuprofen a couple of times a week if the pain is particularly bad; this helps within half an hour.

State of health between attacks

EL reports that she is 'fine' apart from the headaches. Migraines are infrequent and she can cope with them. She is concerned about the daily headaches as she is worried that they may start to affect her work. She feels tired most of the time but sleeps well. In response to the question 'During the last month, have you been bothered by having little interest or pleasure in doing things?' EL replies that she would love to spend time with her friends and go out, but has not had the free time to do so. She has never injured her neck or back and is otherwise fit and well.

Examination

BP 120/80 with a regular pulse of 74 beats per minute. EL looks tired but otherwise well. Funduscopy and brief neurological examination were unremarkable. The trapezius and longus colli muscles on both sides were tender to palpation.

Investigations

As there are no sinister symptoms in the history and no abnormal findings on physical examination, there is no indication for investigations.

ABC of Headache. Edited by A. MacGregor & A. Frith.
© 2009 Blackwell Publishing, ISBN 978-1-4051-7066-6.

Diagnosis

Differential diagnosis

EL has identified two different headaches: recurrent, episodic 'sick' headaches and daily headaches. The only significant clinical sign is pericranial muscle tenderness on palpation. There is no history of depression. There is no evidence of medication overuse in the history, although this will need to be confirmed with prospective diary cards. In the absence of any other clinical signs, primary headaches are likely (Figure 3.1).

Preliminary diagnosis

Although it can sometimes be difficult to differentiate between coexisting headaches, EL already knows that her infrequent headaches are migraine without aura. The clinical features of recurrent, episodic 'sick' headaches confirm this diagnosis.

The probable diagnosis for recurrent daily headaches in an otherwise well person, in the absence of any specific features or clinical signs, is tension-type headache. This is the most common type of primary headache.

Episodic tension-type headache has a one-year prevalence of around 40%. It affects more women than men and peaks in the 20–40 year age groups. It is best defined as 'normal' headaches, which have very little impact on the individual. They occur in attack-like episodes, with variable and often very low frequency, and are mostly short-lasting – no more than several hours. Headache can be unilateral but is more often generalized. It is typically described as pressure or tightness, like a vice or tight band around the head, and commonly spreads into or arises from the neck. Whilst it can be disabling for a few hours, it lacks the specific features and associated symptom complex of migraine (Box 3.1). Tension-type headache is frequently attributed to stress (Table 3.1). Clinically, there are cases where stress is obvious and likely to be aetiologically implicated (often in headache that becomes worse during the day) and others where it is not apparent. It often coexists with migraine without aura, causing diagnostic confusion. Unless both conditions are recognized and managed individually, the outcome is unlikely to be successful.

Chronic tension-type headache is less common, with a one-year prevalence of 2–3%. It typically evolves over time from episodic tension-type headache. It occurs, by definition, on more than 15 days a month, and may be daily (Box 3.2). The chronic subtype is associated with disability and high personal and socio-economic costs.

The exact mechanisms of tension-type headache are not known. Tension-type headache may be stress-related or associated with functional or structural cervical or cranial musculoskeletal abnormality. Increased pericranial tenderness on manual palpation is the most significant abnormal finding in patients with tension-type headache.

Initial management

This includes:
- reassurance
- identification of underlying contributory factors

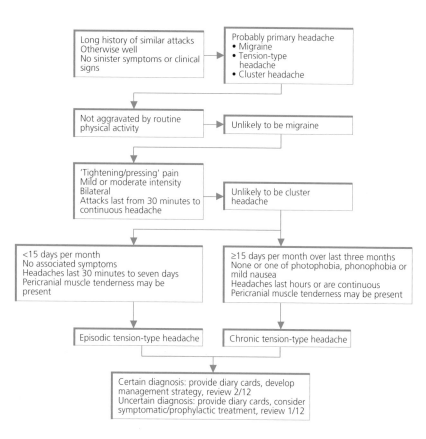

Figure 3.1 Flowchart of differential diagnosis

Box 3.1 **International Classification of Headache Disorders. Diagnostic criteria for episodic tension-type headache**

Diagnostic criteria

A. At least 10 episodes occurring on <1 day a month on average (<12 days a year) and fulfilling criteria B–D (infrequent episodic tension-type headache) OR at least 10 episodes occurring on ≥1 but <15 days per month for at least three months (≥12 and <180 days per year) and fulfilling criteria B–D (frequent episodic tension-type headache)

B. Headache attacks lasting from 30 minutes to seven days

C. Headache has at least two of the following characteristics:
  1. bilateral location
  2. pressing/tightening (non-pulsating) quality
  3. mild or moderate intensity
  4. not aggravated by routine physical activity such as walking or climbing stairs

D. Both of the following:
  1. no nausea or vomiting (anorexia may occur)
  2. no more than one of photophobia or phonophobia

E. Not attributed to another disorder

Note: Episodic tension-type headache may or may not be associated with increased pericranial tenderness on manual palpation.
Source: adapted from Headache Classification Subcommittee of the International Headache Society (IHS). *The International Classification of Headache Disorders* (2nd edition). *Cephalalgia* 2004; **24** (suppl 1): 1–160.

Box 3.2 **International Classification of Headache Disorders. Diagnostic criteria for chronic tension-type headache**

Diagnostic criteria

A. Headache occurring on ≥15 days per month on average for three months (≥180 days a year) and fulfilling criteria B–D

B. Headache lasts hours or may be continuous

C. Headache has at least two of the following characteristics:
  1. bilateral location
  2. pressing/tightening (non-pulsating) quality
  3. mild or moderate intensity
  4. not aggravated by routine physical activity such as walking or climbing stairs

D. Both of the following:
  1. no more than one of photophobia, phonophobia or mild nausea
  2. neither moderate/severe nausea nor vomiting

E. Not attributed to another disorder

Note: Chronic tension-type headache may or may not be associated with increased pericranial tenderness on manual palpation.
Source: adapted from Headache Classification Subcommittee of the International Headache Society (IHS). *The International Classification of Headache Disorders* (2nd edition). *Cephalalgia* 2004; **24** (suppl 1):1–160.

Table 3.1 Frequency of various precipitating factors in tension-type headache

Precipitant	Men (%)	Women (%)
Stress and mental tension	64	77
Smoking (including passive smoking)	34	38
Weather changes	26	28
Alcohol	25	28
Certain foods	5	11
Sexual activity	2	3
Menstruation	–	39

Source: Rasmussen BK. Migraine and tension-type headache in a general population: precipitating factors, female hormones, sleep pattern and relation to lifestyle. *Pain* 1993; **53(1)**: 65–72.

Table 3.2 Pharmacological intervention: symptomatic
Restrict to treatment of infrequent episodic tension-type headache

	Dose	**Max. per 24 hours***
Aspirin	600–900 mg	4000 mg
Diclofenac	50–100 mg	150 mg
Ibuprofen	200–400 mg	2400 mg
Ketoprofen	25–50 mg	150 mg
Naproxen	250–500 mg	1250 mg
Paracetamol	500–1000 mg	4000 mg

*Limit to ≤3 days a week.

- appropriate symptomatic treatment
- diary cards to confirm diagnosis, assess frequency and duration of attacks, and response to symptomatic treatment
- review after 4–8 weeks

Symptomatic treatment

Symptomatic treatment (Table 3.2) is appropriate only for episodic tension-type headache occurring on fewer than two days a week. Over-the-counter analgesics, such as aspirin, ibuprofen or paracetamol, are usually sufficient. However, there is evidence that paracetamol is less effective than aspirin (Figure 3.2); prescription NSAIDs are sometimes indicated. Symptomatic treatment is not recommended for chronic tension-type headache as, if taken regularly more than three days a week, can lead to medication overuse headache.

Prophylactic treatment
Non-pharmacological measures

Tension-type headache is more common in sedentary people (Table 3.3). Although there is little research evidence for efficacy on a pragmatic basis, regular exercise is recommended. Physiotherapy may also be appropriate for musculoskeletal symptoms. Physiotherapy may include massage, mobilization, manipulation and, particularly in those with sedentary lifestyles, correction of posture (Box 3.3).

Biofeedback and relaxation therapy are associated with cognitive changes that benefit chronic tension-type headache.

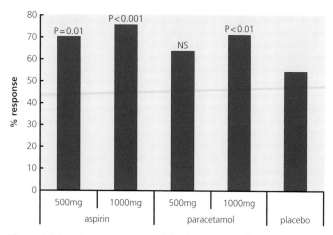

Figure 3.2 Two-hour response rate following treatment for episodic tension-type headache

Source: Steiner TJ, Lange R, Voelker M. Aspirin in episodic tension-type headache: placebo-controlled dose-ranging comparison with paracetamol. *Cephalalgia* 2003; **23(1)**: 59–66.

Box 3.3 **Non-pharmacological intervention**

- Reassurance
- Regular exercise
- Physiotherapy
- Lifestyle changes
    relaxation therapy
    cognitive therapy

Table 3.3 Prevalence rates (%) of tension-type headache according to physical activity at work or as exercise in leisure time

Level of physical activity	Men (%)	Women (%)
Sedentary	33	33
Moderate activity	14	28
Active	14	28
Heavy work/competitive sport	23	40

Source: Rasmussen BK. Migraine and tension-type headache in a general population: precipitating factors, female hormones, sleep pattern and relation to lifestyle. *Pain* 1993; **53(1)**: 65–72.

Pharmacological measures

Amitriptyline is effective and is the treatment of choice for frequent episodic and chronic tension-type headache (Table 3.4 and Figure 3.3). Its use in chronic pain syndromes is not dependent on its antidepressant activity. Side-effects are relatively common but greatly reduced by starting at a low dose (10–25 mg at night). Increments of 10–25 mg should be added as soon as side-effects

Table 3.4 Pharmacological intervention: prophylaxis
For frequent episodic tension-type headache and chronic tension-type headache

Amitriptyline	10–150 mg at night
Mirtazpine	15–30 mg/day
Tizanidine	≤18 mg/day

permit, perhaps each 1–2 weeks and usually into the range 75–150 mg at night. Withdrawal may be attempted after improvement has been maintained for 4–6 months. Nortriptyline and protriptyline may be better tolerated, but have not been as rigorously evaluated.

Failure of tricyclic therapy may be due to sub-therapeutic dosage, insufficient duration of treatment or non-compliance.

Mirtazpine, a noradrenergic and specific serotonergic antidepressant, 15–30 mg/day can be considered for patients who do not respond to amitriptyline. Other antidepressants have not been shown to be effective for tension-type headache in the absence of depression.

Tizanidine, an alpha agonist, has evidence of efficacy for chronic tension-type headache in doses up to 18 mg/day. It should be tried in patients who do not respond to antidepressants.

There is evidence that botulinum toxin is of no benefit.

Management plan

EL acknowledges that her work may be a significant factor in her headaches. She feels that she cannot continue without some effective treatment and starts on amitriptyline 10 mg. She is advised to take this at least two hours before bedtime to limit the sedative effects the next morning. She is made aware that side-effects are worse initially and that she may not experience any benefit in the first couple of weeks. Although she is unable to reduce her working hours, she agrees to return to a regular exercise programme.

Referral

Since there are no sinister features on history or examination, there is no indication to refer EL, unless her symptoms fail to respond to standard management strategies.

Final diagnosis

Eight weeks later, review of EL's diary cards show initial daily headaches with no associated features. She has not taken any symptomatic treatment. This confirms the original diagnosis of chronic tension-type headache. She gradually increased the amitriptyline to 50 mg at night and over the last few weeks has had markedly fewer headaches. She tolerates the amitriptyline well, although initially she experienced dry mouth, sedation and constipation. She has

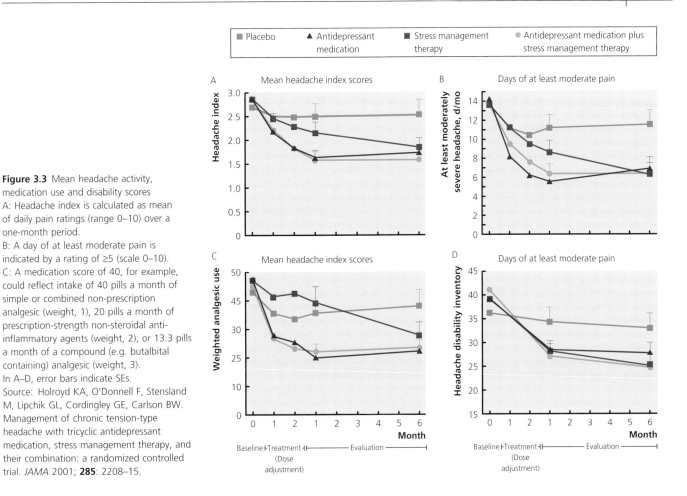

Figure 3.3 Mean headache activity, medication use and disability scores
A: Headache index is calculated as mean of daily pain ratings (range 0–10) over a one-month period.
B: A day of at least moderate pain is indicated by a rating of ≥5 (scale 0–10).
C: A medication score of 40, for example, could reflect intake of 40 pills a month of simple or combined non-prescription analgesic (weight, 1), 20 pills a month of prescription-strength non-steroidal anti-inflammatory agents (weight, 2), or 13.3 pills a month of a compound (e.g. butalbital containing) analgesic (weight, 3).
In A–D, error bars indicate SEs.
Source: Holroyd KA, O'Donnell F, Stensland M, Lipchik GL, Cordingley GE, Carlson BW. Management of chronic tension-type headache with tricyclic antidepressant medication, stress management therapy, and their combination: a randomized controlled trial. *JAMA* 2001; **285**: 2208–15.

been swimming twice a week and is feeling generally better in herself.

Ongoing management

EL is advised to continue her current strategy for a further 2–4 months.

Outcome

EL has responded to reassurance and a combination of pharmacological and lifestyle interventions. She was able to discontinue the amitriptyline after four months of treatment. She has continued to take regular exercise and now works fixed regular hours. She experiences only occasional tension-type headaches as well as her long-standing migraine.

Further reading

Holroyd KA, O'Donnell F, Stensland M, Lipchik GL, Cordingley GE, Carlson BW. Management of chronic tension-type headache with tricyclic antidepressant medication, stress management therapy, and their combination: a randomized controlled trial. *JAMA* 2001; **285**: 2208–15.

Padberg M, de Bruijn SF, de Haan RJ, Tavy DL. Treatment of chronic tension-type headache with botulinum toxin: a double-blind, placebo-controlled clinical trial. *Cephalalgia* 2004; **24(8)**: 675–80.

Rasmussen BK. Migraine and tension-type headache in a general population: precipitating factors, female hormones, sleep pattern and relation to lifestyle. *Pain* 1993; **53(1)**: 65–72.

Schwartz BS, Stewart WF, Simon D, Lipton RB. Epidemiology of tension-type headache. *JAMA* 1998; **279(5)**: 381–3.

Steiner TJ, MacGregor EA, Davies PTG. *Guidelines for All Healthcare Professionals in the Diagnosis and Management of Migraine, Tension-Type, Cluster and Medication Overuse Headache* (3rd edition 2007). www.bash.org.uk

Welch KMA. A 47-year-old woman with tension-type headaches. *JAMA* 2001; **286(8)**: 960–6.

CHAPTER 4

Cluster Headache

David W. Dodick

OVERVIEW

- Cluster headache occurs in both males and females (3:1)
- Cluster headaches are very severe, strictly unilateral, usually last about an hour and may recur up to eight times a day
- Nocturnal attacks are common and obstructive sleep apnoea is a frequent co-morbidity
- Secondary causes must be excluded and differentiation between other trigeminal autonomic cephalalgias has important treatment implications
- Oxygen, parenteral triptans and verapamil are the treatments of choice

CASE HISTORY

The woman with seasonal headaches

EE is 52 years old. She has had stereotyped headaches for 20 years. In recent years, the headaches usually occur 2–4 times a day, every day, for a period of two months during the winter, and then resolve for 8–10 months before returning. She will usually awaken during the night with at least one attack, which occurs at about 2.30 am. Attacks can be triggered by alcohol, but only during the susceptible two-month period. The pain is excruciating, always on the right side and described as a spike in the right eye going through to the occiput. The pain peaks within one minute, and if untreated, lasts about one hour. During this time her right eyelid droops, the right eye tears and becomes red, and she develops nasal drainage on the right. She will always have to pace, walk or even run on the spot to try to distract herself from the pain.

History

How many different headache types does the patient experience?

EE has only one type of headache. When she is not experiencing these severe headaches during the susceptible two-month period, she is free of headaches.

ABC of Headache. Edited by A. MacGregor & A. Frith.
© 2009 Blackwell Publishing, ISBN 978-1-4051-7066-6.

Time questions

The headaches began 20 years ago. Initially, she may have experienced remission periods lasting up to three years, but over the last five years they have been occurring annually. Each painful attack lasts about 60 minutes, and can recur up to four times a day, every day, for two months. In between each attack EE is often free of headache, though she may have a lingering dull ache (a 'shadow' of the last attack) that lasts several hours. She is a lawyer for a large healthcare organization. During this two-month period it is almost impossible for her to continue to work.

Character questions

The character of the pain is knife-like, centred in the right eye, with radiation to the right occiput. The pain is more intense than childbirth according to the patient, who has two children, and on a 10-point pain severity scale, her attacks are 10/10. There is no associated aura, but she does experience ipsilateral photophobia and nausea during the attacks. During every attack she develops ipsilateral conjunctival injection, lacrimation, ptosis and rhinorrhoea.

Cause questions

There are no particular factors which appear to provoke each two-month cluster of attacks other than the season. The attacks usually begin during winter. Alcohol will almost always trigger an attack during a cluster phase, but not during the 8–10-month remission phase. At least one attack will occur each night and awaken her from sleep at about 2.30 am. Her husband reports that he is sometimes awakened by her loud snoring. There is no history of anyone in her family suffering similar attacks.

Response to headache questions

EE must move, pace or jog during these attacks. She cannot sit or lie still. This factor, in addition to the intensity of the pain and her inability to concentrate on anything other than the pain, makes it very difficult to remain at work or to prepare her materials for court. During these two months her professional, personal and social life becomes severely disrupted. She has been treated with antibiotics for a presumed sinus infection without benefit. She has also been treated with propranolol 60 mg daily and amitriptyline 75 mg daily but neither was effective in reducing the frequency or severity of the pain. Oral sumatriptan 50 mg and zolmitriptan 2.5 mg were minimally effective in reducing the severity of the pain. Oral analgesics and opioids have been completely ineffective.

State of health between attacks

After the cluster cycle has resolved, the patient feels completely well. However, during the two-month cycle she feels miserable between attacks, still may have some residual pain and nausea, and becomes very anxious anticipating the next attack, which invariably will strike within four hours after the last attack resolves.

Examination

Vital signs were within normal limits, and general physical and neurological examination was normal except for a mild ptosis of the right eyelid without papillary asymmetry. There are no neck bruits.

Referral

Given the cyclical nature of these symptoms, cluster-like headaches are suspected. Since few primary care physicians have experience of this condition, early referral to a specialist is recommended. If patients are treated in primary care, referral should be considered in those who do not respond to conventional treatment (see below) and/or when such treatments are contraindicated due to coexisting diseases (e.g. cardiovascular disease contraindicates the use of triptans).

Investigations

Electrocardiogram is recommended in all patients who may receive verapamil. EE's ECG was normal with no evidence of heart block.

The specialist referred EE for overnight sleep studies, which revealed obstructive sleep apnoea (OSA) with apnoeic episodes occurring primarily during rapid eye movement (REM) sleep. She experienced a typical attack during an REM-related apnoeic episode associated with oxygen desaturation to 85%. Sleep studies are not a typical investigation but should be considered in patients with cluster-like symptoms as there may be an association with OSA.

MRI of the brain with gadolinium and coronal images through the sella turcica was normal.

Diagnosis

Differential diagnosis

The differential diagnosis includes secondary causes of cluster-like headache and other trigeminal autonomic cephalalgias (TACs) (Table 4.1). The likelihood that a secondary cause is present is quite low given the duration of illness (20 years), the periodicity of attack phases with 8–10-month remission phases and the lack of abnormal neurological signs, except for mild ptosis of the ipsilateral lid. Patients with cluster headache may have residual ptosis or a Horner's syndrome between attacks or even between cluster periods. Nevertheless, brain MRI with coronal cuts through the sella turcica is recommended in patients who present with cluster headache and other trigeminal autonomic cephalalgia to exclude the presence of a pituitary lesion (e.g. adenoma) or parasellar mass that may be slow growing. If no secondary cause is identified, then the

Table 4.1 Distinguishing features of cluster headache and other trigeminal autonomic cephalalgias

Feature	PH	SUNCT	Cluster
Sex F:M	2:1	1:2	1:3
Attack duration (mean)	~15 mins	~1 min	60 mins
Attack frequency per 24 hours (mean)	11	~30	1
Treatment of choice	Indometacin	Lamotrigine	Verapamil

PH: Paroxysmal hemicrania, SUNCT: Short-lasting unilateral neuralgiform headache attacks with conjunctival injection and tearing.

> **Box 4.1 International Classification of Headache Disorders. Diagnostic criteria for cluster headache**
>
> *Diagnostic criteria*
> A. At least five attacks fulfilling criteria B–D
> B. Severe or very severe unilateral orbital, supraorbital and/or temporal pain lasting 15–180 minutes if untreated
> C. Headache is accompanied by at least one of the following:
> 1. ipsilateral conjunctival injection and/or lacrimation
> 2. ipsilateral nasal congestion and/or rhinorrhoea
> 3. ipsilateral eyelid oedema
> 4. ipsilateral forehead and facial sweating
> 5. ipsilateral miosis and/or ptosis
> 6. a sense of restlessness or agitation
> D. Attacks have a frequency from one every other day to eight per day
> E. Not attributed to another disorder
>
> Source: Headache Classification Subcommittee of the International Headache Society (IHS). *The International Classification of Headache Disorders* (2nd edition). *Cephalalgia* 2004; **24** (suppl 1): 1–160.

differentiation of episodic cluster headache from episodic paroxysmal hemicrania (EPH) and short-lasting unilateral neuralgiform headache attacks with conjunctival injection and tearing (SUNCT) syndrome is important since the treatments for each are different.

Preliminary diagnosis

Episodic cluster headache is the diagnosis (Box 4.1). Brain MRI revealed no intracranial lesions and overnight polysomnogram revealed REM-related OSA, which was associated with a typical cluster attack. The attack frequency (2–4 attacks per 24 hours) and duration of each attack (approximately one hour) are most compatible with cluster headache. While the attack phenotype associated with EPH (Box 4.2) and SUNCT (Box 4.3) may be identical – severe, strictly unilateral pain with cranial autonomic features such as lacrimation, conjunctival injection and rhinorrhoea – the 24-hour attack frequency is higher with both of these disorders and the attack duration is shorter (Figures 4.1 and 4.2). The presence of photophobia and nausea during attacks illustrates the potential for symptoms that are believed to be characteristic of migraine to occur during cluster attacks. The ipsilateral nature of the photophobia may be a useful distinguishing feature between migraine and cluster headache in particular, and the TACs in general. The agitation during each attack is also characteristic of cluster headache and a further feature that distinguishes this disorder from migraine, where patients usually prefer to be still and supine.

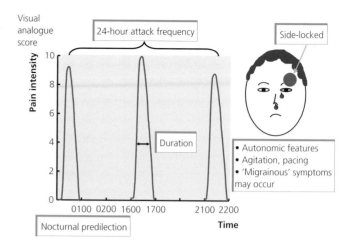

Figure 4.1 Cardinal clinical characteristics of cluster headache
Source: Cittadini E, Goadsby PG. Paroxysmal hemicrania: a case series of twenty-five patients. *Neurology* 2007; **68**: A89–A90.

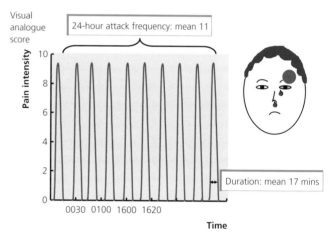

Figure 4.2 Paroxysmal hemicrania: features that differentiate from cluster headache
Source: Cittadini E, Goadsby PG. Paroxysmal hemicrania: a case series of twenty-five patients. *Neurology* 2007; **68**: A89–A90.

Initial management

This includes:
- avoidance of triggers (high altitude, nitrates, alcohol)
- treatment of obstructive sleep apnoea
- acute symptomatic treatment
- transitional prophylactic treatment
- maintenance prophylactic treatment

Acute symptomatic treatment

Acute treatment of cluster headache must ensure rapid relief of pain. The pain is very severe, peaks rapidly and lasts for a relatively short time (mean 60 minutes). Therefore, oral medications do not provide sufficiently rapid relief of pain. The most effective treatments include high-flow 100% oxygen at a rate of 7–15 L per minute, through a non re-breathing face mask, subcutaneous sumatriptan 6 mg and intranasal sumatriptan 20 mg or zolmitriptan 10 mg. Recently, a European Consensus Statement provided

Table 4.2 Evidence-based acute treatment recommendations for trigeminal autonomic cephalalgias

Therapy	Treatment of choice		
	Cluster headache	Paroxysmal hemicrania	SUNCT syndrome
Acute	100% O$_2$, 15 L/min (A) Sumatriptan 6 mg s.c. (A) Sumatriptan 20 mg nasal (A) Zolmitriptan 10 mg nasal (A) Zolmitriptan 10 mg oral (B) Lidocaine nasal (B) Octreotide (B)	None	None

A = effective, B = probably effective.
Source: EFNS Guidelines. May A, et al., *Eur J Neurol* 2006; **13(10)**: 1066–77.

Table 4.3 Evidence-based preventive treatment recommendations for trigeminal autonomic cephalalgias

Therapy	Treatment of choice		
	Cluster headache	Paroxysmal hemicrania	SUNCT syndrome
Preventive	Verapamil (A) Corticosteroids (A) (orally/occipital nerve block)* Lithium carbonate (B) Methysergide (B) Topiramate (B) Ergotamine tartrate (B) Valproic acid (C) Melatonin (C) Gabapentin (C)*	Indometacin (A) Verapamil (C) NSAIDs (C)	Topiramate (B)* Lamotrigine (C) Gabapentin (C)*

*Adapted.
A = effective, B = probably effective, C = possibly effective.
Source: EFNS Guidelines. May A, et al., *Eur J Neurol* 2006; **13(10)**: 1066–77.

evidence-based recommendations for the acute and preventive treatment of cluster headache (Table 4.2).

Transitional prophylactic treatment

This treatment strategy refers to the use of a therapy that will induce rapid suppression of the attacks for a period of 1–2 weeks. The rationale for this treatment strategy is to eliminate or reduce the frequency of attacks during the time that it usually takes for maintenance prophylactic therapies to exert their efficacy. This strategy should obviate the need for the repetitive use of acute treatments several times a day. The most frequent transitional strategy is oral corticosteroids. Ipsilateral greater occipital nerve blockade is increasingly used. While there is no standardized regimen for the use of oral corticosteroids, one frequently used regimen includes the use of prednisolone 60 mg for 2–3 days, with 10 mg decrements every 2–3 days (e.g. 50 mg for 2–3 days, 40 mg for 2–3 days, etc.).

Maintenance prophylactic treatment

The drug of first choice for the maintenance prevention of cluster headache is verapamil. The dosage range is 240–960 mg in three divided daily dosages. In some patients higher than conventional dosages may be required (>480 mg per day) for efficacy. Periodic monitoring of electrocardiograms over the course of therapy is important since heart block may occur in up to 10% of patients, even after long periods of treatment where the drug is seemingly well tolerated. The drug is usually used for the typical duration of the cluster period, which in EE's case would be two months, plus an additional period until the patient is completely attack-free for two weeks. Other preventive medications and the level of evidence are outlined in Table 4.3.

Final diagnosis

Episodic cluster headache. EE preferred an intranasal triptan, with which she experienced relief within 10 minutes and became pain-free within 20 minutes. Cluster attacks resolved within 48 hours of starting oral prednisolone, and verapamil was titrated up to a dose

of 120 mg three times a day. Treatment was continued for 10 weeks, and then gradually decreased by 120 mg every five days.

Management plan

The patient was given prescriptions for oral prednisolone, intranasal zolmitriptan and verapamil. These prescriptions were to be filled at the onset of her next cluster cycle, at which point she was encouraged to call the office for a follow-up visit. She was also encouraged to use a nasal continuous positive airway pressure (CPAP) device to treat her OSA.

Outcome

The outcome associated with this cluster cycle was positive. EE became attack-free within 48 hours, during which time she was able to manage attacks effectively with intranasal zolmitriptan, and remained attack-free for the next two months. Thus far, there is no evidence that long-term maintenance therapy is effective in reducing the next cluster cycle. In addition, patients with cluster headache may experience long-term remission and for these reasons, it is generally considered prudent to taper and discontinue preventive treatments between cluster cycles.

Further reading

Cohen AS, Matharu MS, Goadsby PJ. Trigeminal autonomic cephalalgias: current and future treatments. *Headache* 2007; **47(6)**: 969–80.

Cohen AS, Matharu MS, Goadsby PJ. Electrocardiographic abnormalities in patients with cluster headache on verapamil therapy. *Neurology* 2007; **69(7)**: 668–75.

May A, Leone M, Afra J, Linde M, Sandor PS, Evers S, Goadsby PJ. EFNS guidelines on the treatment of cluster headache and other trigeminal-autonomic cephalalgias. *Eur J Neurol* 2006; **13(10)**: 1066–77.

CHAPTER 5

Medication Overuse Headache

David W. Dodick

OVERVIEW

- Medication overuse headache is the most common secondary cause of chronic daily headache (headache >15 days/month)
- Medication overuse headache occurs most commonly in patients with a prior history of migraine
- The treatment response to withdrawal, short- and long-term prognosis and relapse rates depend on the class of drug overused and the prior headache type
- Preventive migraine therapy is effective for the treatment of medication overuse headache and should be initiated immediately

---

CASE HISTORY

The woman with headaches on most days

TR is a 42-year-old woman presenting with severe episodic migraine occurring approximately four times a month. These attacks are unilateral, on alternate sides, are severe in intensity and are associated with exquisite photophobia, nausea and occasionally emesis. Oral sumatriptan 100 mg provides relief for about 50% of attacks within three hours, but the headache may recur several times over the next 48 hours. She also has a background headache that is present at least 20 days a month. This headache is generalized, bilateral and associated with occipital-nuchal discomfort. It is partially relieved by a combination analgesic (aspirin 325 mg, acetaminophen 325 mg, caffeine 65 mg).

History

How many different headache types does the patient experience?

TR believes she has two types of headache. The first is what she feels is a typical migraine attack which occurs four times a month. The second is a background generalized headache that is present at least 20 days a month. She has only about 3–5 headache-free days a month.

ABC of Headache. Edited by A. MacGregor & A. Frith.
© 2009 Blackwell Publishing, ISBN 978-1-4051-7066-6.

Time questions

TR has a history of migraine without aura which began during menarche. Migraine attacks were quite infrequent until she attended university, when she began to develop more frequent attacks (3–4 a month). Without an obvious precipitating factor, her migraine attacks continued to increase in frequency, her use of acute medications increased, and over the course of 1–2 years she developed near-daily headache. While her headaches used to occur in relation to her menstrual cycle, she had an abdominal hysterectomy for uterine fibroids two years ago.

Character questions

The pain associated with each migraine attack is severe, bursting in quality and involves the entire half of her head, from the occiput to the periorbital region. Each attack is associated with premonitory nausea. Pain is worsened by routine physical activity and associated with severe photophobia and osmophobia. She vomits with at least 25% of attacks. The headache may return after initial relief, and the duration of each attack ranges from 12 to 48 hours. The milder headache is dull, aching and generalized. She is mildly photophobic with these headaches, but experiences no other symptoms.

Cause questions

The most common trigger factors for a migraine attack are sleep deprivation, stressful life events, alcohol and strong odours such as perfume. They are partially responsive to rest, cold cloth binding the head and oral sumatriptan. There are no particular triggers for the background near-daily headache other than anxiety or anticipation that she will develop a migraine attack prior to an important meeting or social event. Her mother, sister and daughter suffer from migraine. Her mother used to experience near-daily headache as well, but both types of headache appeared to diminish after menopause.

Response to headache questions

TR is usually disabled during migraine attacks. She will have to rest after taking her triptan but can sometimes remain at work and perform her duties, with difficulty, as an administrative assistant. The daily headache does not keep her from work, but she feels it certainly reduces her performance at times when it becomes moderately severe. She misses about 2–5 days of work each month, and her employer has expressed dissatisfaction with her frequent absences. She will frequently avoid scheduling social and leisure activities and often misses family activities. She uses 12 oral sumatriptan 100 mg tablets a month, usually two tablets per attack across six treatment days. She also uses a combination analgesic (aspirin 325 mg, acetaminophen 325 mg, caffeine 65 mg) approximately 20 days a month, with an average of four per day.

State of health between attacks

TR is seldom without headache and some degree of photophobia and/or nausea. She is increasingly anxious about the next severe disabling migraine attack, which prompts her to treat the background headache frequently to prevent it from 'growing' into a migraine attack. She is becoming increasingly depressed, feels inadequate as a wife and mother, cannot participate fully in family activities and is concerned about losing her job due to frequent absences related to headache and reduced work productivity.

Examination

Affect was blunted and mood was depressed. The patient appeared anxious. Vital signs were within normal limits, and general physical and neurological examination was normal. Body mass index was 23. Musculoskeletal examination revealed mild tenderness over the posterior skull base, cervical paraspinal and trapezius muscles. Range of motion of the cervical spine was, however, normal. No evidence of papilloedema.

Investigations

Complete blood count and serum chemistry were normal. No evidence for anaemia or renal insufficiency.

Diagnosis

Differential diagnosis

The history is of episodic migraine transforming gradually to near-daily headache commensurate with increasing use of acute headache medications. The overall duration of illness and normal examination are not consistent with an underlying organic secondary cause other than acute medication overuse. While the background daily headache is often attributed to tension-type headache, daily diary studies have demonstrated that most headache days in patients with medication overuse headache (MOH) meet International Classification of Headache Disorders (ICHD-II) criteria for migraine or probable migraine. While this patient appears to meet ICHD-II diagnostic criteria for chronic migraine, the presence of medication overuse precludes this diagnosis at the time of consultation, at least as long as medication overuse is present.

Preliminary diagnosis

Medication overuse headache. The diagnostic criteria for MOH have recently been defined by the International Headache Society (Boxes 5.1 and 5.2). In practice, MOH should be suspected when:
- headache is present on ≥15 days per month
- regular overuse of >3 months of one or more acute medications
- headache has developed or markedly worsened during medication overuse.

Box 5.1 International Classification of Headache Disorders. Diagnostic criteria for triptan overuse headache

Diagnostic criteria
A. Headache present on >15 days/month with at least one of the following characteristics and fulfilling criteria C and D:
  1. predominantly unilateral
  2. pulsating quality
  3. moderate or severe intensity
  4. aggravated by or causing avoidance of routine physical activity (e.g. walking or climbing stairs)
  5. associated with at least one of the following:
    a) nausea and/or vomiting
    b) photophobia and phonophobia
B. Triptan intake (any formulation) on ≥10 days/month on a regular basis for ≥3 months
C. Headache frequency has markedly increased during triptan overuse
D. Headache reverts to its previous pattern within two months after discontinuation of triptan

Source: Headache Classification Subcommittee of the International Headache Society (IHS). *The International Classification of Headache Disorders* (2nd edition). *Cephalalgia* 2004; **24** (suppl 1): 1–160.

Box 5.2 International Classification of Headache Disorders. Diagnostic criteria for analgesic overuse headache

Diagnostic criteria
A. Headache present on >15 days/month with at least one of the following characteristics and fulfilling criteria C and D:
  1. bilateral
  2. pressing/tightening (non-pulsating) quality
  3. mild or moderate intensity
B. Intake of simple analgesics on ≥15 days/month for >3 months
C. Headache has developed or markedly worsened during analgesic overuse
D. Headache resolves or reverts to its previous pattern within two months after discontinuation of analgesics

Source: Headache Classification Subcommittee of the International Headache Society (IHS). *The International Classification of Headache Disorders* (2nd edition). *Cephalalgia* 2004; **24** (suppl 1): 1–160.

MOH can result from most acute medications used for relief of headache, but the threshold for causing MOH differs depending on the class of medication that is overused (Box 5.3).

Initial management

This includes:
- avoidance of migraine triggers
- abrupt cessation of triptans and combination analgesic
- acute symptomatic treatment of moderate or severe headache only
- strict limits on the frequency of acute medication use (≤2 days per week)

Box 5.3 **Threshold for each class of medication for the diagnosis of medication overuse headache**

- Ergot, triptan, opioid or butalbital analgesics
  Taken on a regular basis ≥10 days/month
- Other analgesics
  Non-opioid analgesics ≥15 days/month
- Total exposure
  Two or more acute drugs ≥15 days/month

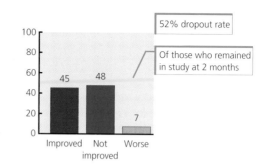

Figure 5.1 Short-term outcomes in patients undergoing withdrawal alone without preventive therapy.
Source: adapted from Zeeberg P, Olesen J, Jensen R. Probable medication-overuse headche: the effect of 2-month drug-free period. *Neurology* 2006; **66**: 1894–8.

- initiation of preventive medication
- employment of non-pharmacological strategies when indicated (e.g. biofeedback, relaxation therapy)

Acute symptomatic treatment

Acute treatment of withdrawal headaches and migraine attacks must be provided to minimize suffering and maximize compliance. The preferred acute treatments are non-steroidal anti-inflammatory medications (NSAIDs) and/or dihydroergotamine (DHE), if available. Dihydroergotamine can be delivered by intranasal, subcutaneous or intramuscular routes of administration. These medications are considered to have a very low propensity for inducing MOH and are effective for the acute treatment of migraine. Their use, however, should be limited to two treatment days a week. It is recommended that combination analgesics and opioids be avoided. Triptans may be used for acute symptomatic relief of moderate or severe migraine attacks or withdrawal headaches, so long as a triptan was not one of the overused medications that have been withdrawn.

Initiation of preventive medication

It is recommended that preventive medication be initiated immediately, especially since withdrawal alone is effective in less than 50% of patients (Figure 5.1).

Topiramate has been shown to reduce headache frequency, migraine frequency and consumption of acute medications in patients with MOH even when the acute medications have not been withdrawn or tapered. Preventive medications may also reduce the severity of withdrawal headaches, increase compliance with the withdrawal protocol and reduce the likelihood of relapse or recidivism. Only recently have placebo-controlled studies been conducted in patients with MOH using preventive medications. The only preventive medication to have demonstrated efficacy at this point is topiramate, though from a clinical standpoint, preventive medications with evidence for efficacy in the treatment of episodic migraine may be used. Some authorities recommend naproxen, 250 mg tds or 500 mg bd, taken regularly whether symptoms are present or not, which also pre-empts acute treatment. The purpose of this instruction is to break the habit of responding to pain with medication. Naproxen should be prescribed for a course of 3–4 weeks, and not repeated; some specialists suggest it is taken three times daily for two weeks, twice daily for two weeks, once daily for two weeks and then stopped. Prednisolone, 60 mg/day for two days, 40 mg/day for two days and

20 mg/day for two days, has also been used. An alternative is to start amitriptyline, 10–75 mg at night, which is then continued as long-term prophylaxis.

Referral

Referral should be considered in the patient with significant psychiatric co-morbidity, opioid, barbiturate or benzodiazepine overuse, or when initial attempts at outpatient withdrawal have failed despite the use of preventive treatment.

Final diagnosis

Medication overuse headache.

Management plan

TR abruptly discontinued the combination analgesic and sumatriptan. Topiramate was initiated at a dose of 25 mg a day and increased to 50 mg bd over the course of four weeks. Intranasal dihydroergotamine 2 mg was used for acute symptomatic relief of moderate or severe headache with a limit of two treatment days (4 mg) a week. DHE was used in combination with metoclopramide 10 mg to prevent nausea and enhance the efficacy of DHE. TR was scheduled for a consultation with a neuropsychologist to provide behavioural and non-pharmacological strategies (biofeedback, relaxation therapy) to reduce pain and suffering and to enhance compliance with and effectiveness of the pharmacological strategies initiated.

Outcome

Two months after treatment was initiated, TR's migraine frequency declined to three attacks a month, with each treated effectively with a combination of intranasal DHE plus metoclopramide 10 mg. Topiramate was continued at a dose of 50 mg bd.

Prognosis

The prognosis of MOH depends on the medication being overused and the prior headache type (Figure 5.2). The prognosis is more favourable for patients with migraine, compared to tension-type headache. The short- and long-term prognosis is also more

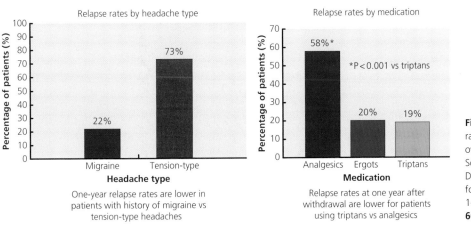

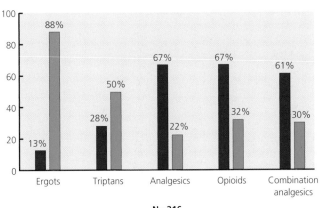

Figure 5.2 Long-term prognosis and relapse rates depend on class of acute medication overused and prior headache type
Source: Katsarava Z, Limmroth V, Finke M, Diener HC, Fritsche G. Rates and predictors for relapse in medication overuse headache: a 1-year prospective study. *Neurology* 2003; **60(10)**: 1682–3.

Figure 5.3 Short-term prognosis and outcomes after withdrawal depends on class of acute medication overused
Source: Adapted from Zeeberg P, Olesen J, Jensen R. Probable medication-overuse headache: the effect of a 2-month drug-free period. *Neurology* 2006; **66**: 1894–8.

favourable when triptans or ergots are overused compared to analgesics, combination analgesics or opioids (Figure 5.3).

Further reading

Katsarava Z, Jensen R. Medication-overuse headache: where are we now? *Curr Opin in Neurol* 2007; **20(3)**: 326–30.

Katsarava Z, Limmroth V, Finke M, Diener HC, Fritsche G. Rates and predictors for relapse in medication overuse headache: a 1-year prospective study. *Neurology* 2003; **60(10)**: 1682–3.

Silberstein SD, Lipton RB, Saper JR. Chronic daily headache including transformed migraine, chronic tension-type headache, and medication overuse headache. In *Wolff's Headache* (8th edition). Eds Stephen D. Silberstein, Richard B. Lipton, David W. Dodick. Oxford and New York: Oxford University Press, 2007.

Zeeberg P, Olesen J, Jensen R. Probable medication-overuse headache: the effect of a 2-month drug-free period. *Neurology* 2006; **66**:1894–8.

CHAPTER 6

Menstrual Headaches

Alison Frith

OVERVIEW

- Fifty per cent of women with migraine report an association with menstruation
- Menstrual migraine is more severe and difficult to treat than non-menstrual migraine in some women
- Diary cards are essential for accurate diagnosis as there are no specific investigations
- Standard acute treatments are the same as for non-menstrual attacks
- Specific prophylaxis for menstrual migraine must be individualized and may be perimenstrual or continuous, contraceptive or non-hormonal

CASE HISTORY

The woman with menstrual headaches
ET is a 39-year-old office worker. She presents with a severe headache occurring either just before or at the start of menstruation each month. She often wakes with pulsating pain, mainly in the right temple. She always feels nauseous and may vomit. She has to lie down and is missing time from work. The headache lasts 2–3 days. Unlike her other headaches occurring once or twice at other times of the month, this headache does not respond to over-the-counter analgesia. ET dreads her period because she is 'struck down' each month. The menstrual headache is the reason for the consultation.

History

How many different headache types does the patient experience?

ET describes two types of headaches: mild headaches at any time during her menstrual cycle, and severe menstrual headaches at the start of menses each month.

Time questions

ET remembers having headaches since her early teens. When she was taking the combined hormonal contraceptive pill she noticed headaches were mainly during the pill-free interval. Headaches

were absent during pregnancy. Headaches occurred 1–3 times a month for up to a day at a time, sometimes with menstruation, and usually responded to over-the-counter analgesia. She has noticed the severe headache with menstruation in the last year.

Character questions

ET describes non-menstrual headaches as a mild-to-moderate pulsating pain felt mainly in her right temple but which can occur in the left temple and/or switch sides. Moving exacerbates the pain, while keeping still helps. ET feels nauseous and is sensitive to light, sound and smell. There are no warning signs or visual symptoms and these headaches tend to build up over the course of a day. ET's menstrual headache is similar but much more severe and debilitating and may be present on waking. Vomiting usually occurs several times over the three-day duration of a bad attack.

Cause questions

ET's non-menstrual headaches can occur without recognized causes, but she has identified being tired, stressed, travelling, missing meals and drinking alcohol as triggers. ET thinks that her menstrual headaches are caused by hormone imbalances. 'Women's headaches' at period time run in the family: her mother used to experience menstrual headaches until her menopause, when the headaches stopped.

Response to headache questions

Non-menstrual headaches do not stop ET from her usual activities; however, she is missing time from work with the menstrual headache. She avoids light and noise, and has to lie down. Severe pain and vomiting make her weak and she feels debilitated for several days afterwards.

State of health between attacks

With no significant past medical history ET was well, apart from feeling slightly more tired than usual. Her periods are regular every 29–31 days. Menstrual flow has been heavier and associated with abdominal cramps in the past six months. ET did not report any symptoms of premenstrual syndrome. She only takes analgesia for headaches and dysmenorrhoea. Losing time with the severe menstrual headache and associated symptoms has begun to worry ET. She is anxious about missing work and fearful of making plans at period time.

ABC of Headache. Edited by A. MacGregor & A. Frith.
© 2009 Blackwell Publishing, ISBN 978-1-4051-7066-6.

Examination

ET is normotensive. There are no abnormal findings on funduscopy, medical or neurological examination.

Investigations

The headache history and examination do not suggest the need for investigations. ET asked about hormone tests, but these are not helpful in diagnosing or treating menstrual headaches. No biochemical or hormonal abnormalities have been found compared to control groups; women with menstrual headaches appear more sensitive to normal hormonal fluctuations.

If ET's menstrual flow remains heavy and tiredness persists, anaemia should be excluded. If menstrual problems continue, then further investigation, including referral to a gynaecologist, may be warranted.

Diagnosis

Differential diagnosis

Headache is a common feature of menstrual disorders, but specific diagnosis of the headache is important. For ET there is no evidence of medication overuse headache or daily headaches, but this would need to be confirmed with diary records. Her two headaches are similar, but the menstrual one is much more severe. Absence of clinical signs for either suggests that these are primary headaches. Tension-type headaches are typically bilateral, have a pressing or tightening quality and are not usually associated with specific symptoms such as nausea. ET's headaches are unilateral, have a pulsating quality and have associated symptoms so migraine is the most likely diagnosis.

Preliminary diagnosis

All ET's headaches fulfil the International Headache Society (IHS) criteria for migraine without aura (Box 6.1). Migraine is more prevalent in women (Figure 6.1). In some women hormonal changes can be a trigger for migraine and this includes the changes at menstruation (Box 6.2).

Migraine without aura in menstruating women that is frequently associated with menses is 'menstrual migraine'. The IHS classifies this general term in two sub-types to allow further scientific study and validation (Box 6.3). Menstrual attacks are usually without aura, even in women who have attacks with aura at other times of the cycle. Pure menstrual migraine is relatively rare compared to menstrually-related migraine (Figure 6.2).

The causes of menstrual migraine are not known. Various possible mechanisms are likely to be a combination of hormonal and neurochemical changes (Figure 6.3). ET's heavy, painful periods suggest prostaglandin release may be a contributory factor as this is known to cause headaches and nausea. ET's history of headaches during the pill-free interval when taking the combined hormonal contraceptive pill, and relative headache freedom during pregnancy, suggest she may be sensitive to oestrogen withdrawal. Oestrogen withdrawal may trigger migraine at menstruation in some women but as prolonged exposure may be required, migraine does

---

Box 6.1 International Classification of Headache Disorders. Diagnostic criteria for migraine without aura

Diagnostic criteria

A. At least five attacks, with one fulfilling criteria B–D
B. Headache attacks lasting 4–72 hours (untreated or unsuccessfully treated)
C. Headache has at least two of the following characteristics:
   1. unilateral location
   2. pulsating quality
   3. moderate or severe pain intensity
   4. aggravation by or causing avoidance of routine physical activity (e.g. walking or climbing stairs)
D. During headache at least one of the following:
   1. nausea and/or vomiting
   2. photophobia and phonophobia
E. Not attributed to another disorder

Source: Headache Classification Subcommittee of the International Headache Society (IHS). *The International Classification of Headache Disorders* (2nd edition). *Cephalalgia* 2004; **24** (suppl 1): 1–160.

Box 6.2 Hormonal associations for migraine

- Migraine has the same prevalence in boys and girls until puberty
- Incidence of migraine increases in girls with the onset of puberty
- Overall migraine is three times more common in women than in men during reproductive years
- Many women with migraine report an association with menses
- Many women experience migraine in the pill-free week when using the combined oral contraceptive pill
- Up to 70% of migraine patients have respite from migraine during pregnancy
- Prevalence of migraine increases in the years leading to menopause
- Migraine often improves or stops after the menopause
- Hormone replacement therapy can help or exacerbate migraine

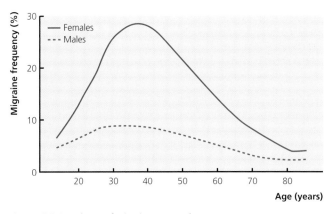

Figure 6.1 Prevalence of migraine: age and sex
Source: Lipton RB, Stewart WF, Diamond S, Diamond ML, Reed M, Prevalence and burden of migraine in the United States: data from the American Migraine Study II. *Headache* 2001; **41**: 646–57.

Box 6.3 **International Classification of Headache Disorders. Diagnostic criteria for menstrual migraine**

Pure menstrual migraine without aura
Diagnostic criteria
A. Attacks in a menstruating woman, fulfilling criteria for migraine without aura (Box 6.1)
B. Attacks occur exclusively on day 1 ± 2 (i.e. days −2 to +3)[1] of menstruation[2] in at least two out of three menstrual cycles and *at no other times* of the cycle

Menstrually-related migraine without aura
Diagnostic criteria
A. Attacks in a menstruating woman, fulfilling criteria for migraine without aura (Box 6.1)
B. Attacks occur on day 1 ± 2 (i.e. days −2 to +3)[1] of menstruation[2] in at least two out of three menstrual cycles and *additionally* at other times of the cycle

Notes:
1. The first day of menstruation is day 1 and the preceding day is day −1; there is no day 0.
2. For the purposes of this classification, menstruation is considered to be endometrial bleeding resulting from either the normal menstrual cycle or from the withdrawal of exogenous progestogens, as in the case of combined oral contraceptives and cyclical hormone replacement therapy.

Source: Headache Classification Subcommittee of the International Headache Society (IHS). *The International Classification of Headache Disorders* (2nd edition). *Cephalalgia* 2004; **24** (suppl 1): 1–160.

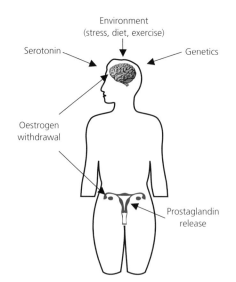

Figure 6.3 Possible mechanisms for menstrual migraine

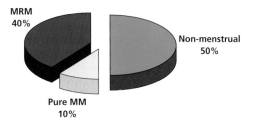
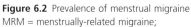

Figure 6.2 Prevalence of menstrual migraine
MRM = menstrually-related migraine;
MM = menstrual migraine
Source: Couturier EGM, Bomhof MAM, Knuistingh Neven A, van Duijn NP. Menstrual migraine in a representative Dutch population sample: prevalence, disability and treatment. *Cephalalgia* 2003; **23**: 302–8; MacGregor EA, Chia H, Vohrah RC, Wilkinson M. Migraine and menstruation: a pilot study. *Cephalalgia* 1990; **10**: 305–10

not occur at ovulation. Oestrogen levels are high during pregnancy and may offer protection against migraine, but they drop during the pill-free interval and in the late luteal phase of the normal menstrual cycle. Declining progesterone levels do not appear to be a migraine trigger factor.

ET's preliminary diagnosis is menstrually-related migraine without aura (Figure 6.4).

Initial management

The initial management strategy is summarized in Box 6.4.

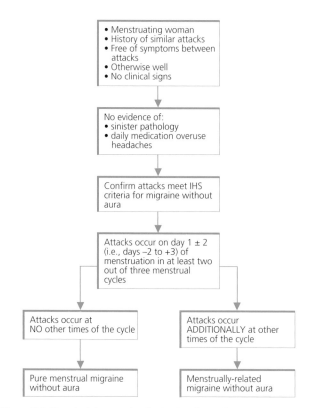

Figure 6.4 Flowchart for menstrual migraine diagnosis

Symptomatic treatment

Menstrual attacks of migraine may be less responsive to treatments; relapse of symptoms is common. There is no difference in symptomatic treatments for menstrual and non-menstrual migraine attacks. Clinical studies have shown that all the triptans available are effective for treating menstrual attacks. For migraine attacks occurring at or around period time, ET was commenced on sumatriptan 50 mg.

Non-pharmacological prevention

ET was encouraged to eliminate non-hormonal triggers. This may improve migraine overall as hormonal and non-hormonal triggers may combine to cause migraines. Remaining hormonally triggered attacks may then respond better to hormonal treatment strategies.

Pharmacological prevention

Diary records showing migraines over three menstrual cycles should be reviewed before considering prophylaxis. This may be

---

Box 6.4 **Initial management of menstrual migraine**

- Confirm migraine diagnosis from history and examination
- If necessary, provide reassurance that treatments are available
- Optimize migraine symptomatic treatment (which may be sufficient)
- Discuss all trigger factors for all migraines and try to eliminate non-hormonal triggers
- Commence headache diary to confirm menstrual migraine diagnosis sub-type, frequency and duration of attacks and response to treatment
- Record each day of menstruation on diary card to assess predictability of menstruation and relationship of headache with menstrual cycle. This may be important for future preventive strategies
- Assess contraceptive requirements which may influence choice of preventive strategy
- Return for review after three complete menstrual cycles

---

perimenstrual or continuous, contraceptive or non-hormonal, and must be based on individual needs, which may change over time. The initial strategy for ET was to optimize acute treatment and consider specific prophylaxis at follow-up if necessary.

Surgical treatment

ET asked if having a hysterectomy could stop her menstrual headaches. It was explained that removing the uterus was only eliminating the end organ and migraine could deteriorate. Also, as migraine often improves after menopause, surgery is not recommended unless there are other medical reasons.

Referral

There is no requirement to refer ET with this headache history. Non-response to standard migraine management strategies may warrant referral to a headache clinic.

Final diagnosis

Three months later at follow-up, ET's diary cards confirm menstrually-related migraine without aura. She has predictable menses (Figure 6.5).

Management plan

ET's non-menstrual migraines were less frequent by avoiding dehydration and long periods without eating. Sumatriptan 50 mg was partially effective for the menstrual attacks, but they relapsed over

---

the City of London

Migraine Clinic

YEAR: *2007*　　NAME: *E.T.*　　DOB: *15/02/1968*

Symptomatic drugs: *Sumatriptan 50 mg, aspirin 300 mg*
Daily prophylactic drugs: *none*
Hormones: *none*
Other regular medication: *none*

	1	2	3	4	5	6	7	8	9	10	11	12	13	14	15	16	17	18	19	20	21	22	23	24	25	26	27	28	29	30	31
January																															
February																															
March																															
April																															
May																															
June																															
July												⊠	⊠	⊠	o	o							X								
August			X							X	⊠	o	⊠	o	o																
September											⊠	⊠	o	o	o						X										
October	X							X	⊠	o	⊠	o	o																		
November																															
December																															

O = period　o = spotting　X = migraine　/ = headache

Figure 6.5 Menstrual migraine diary card

Box 6.5 **Prophylactic strategies for menstrual migraine**

- Consider if symptomatic treatment alone is not effective
- Check that the woman is happy to consider prophylaxis and does not have unreasonable expectations
- Standard migraine prophylaxis is useful when non-menstrual migraine is also a problem
- Co-morbid conditions such as hypertension, depression and epilepsy may influence choice of standard prophylactics
- Diary records are essential to plan treatments and assess effectiveness
- No prophylaxis is licensed for menstrual migraine; clinical trial evidence of efficacy is limited
- A perimenstrual or a continuous strategy will depend on the individual woman
- Prophylaxis should be tried for at least three full menstrual cycles to assess efficacy; women should be counselled to persist for this duration

---

Box 6.6 **Managing menstrual migraine in women who also have migraine with aura**

- Menstrual migraine is typically without aura
- Attacks of migraine with aura typically occur at other times of the cycle
- Contraceptive synthetic oestrogens are contraindicated in women with migraine with aura due to increased risk of ischaemic stroke
- There is no contraindication to physiological doses of natural oestrogens used for perimenstrual oestrogen supplements or hormone replacement therapy
- There is no contraindication to use of progestogen-only strategies

---

several days. The management plan for ET's menstrually-related migraine attacks was to improve acute treatment by increasing the sumatriptan to 100 mg and to start specific prophylaxis.

Prophylactic treatment

Prophylactic treatment specifically for menstrual migraine attacks may be effective for some women, but none is licensed for the indication and clinical trial evidence of efficacy is limited. Few women require specific prophylaxis and there are various considerations (Box 6.5). If migraine aura is present in non-menstrual attacks, contraceptive synthetic oestrogens are contraindicated due to increased risk of ischaemic stroke, but other strategies may be considered (Box 6.6). Perimenstrual or continuous options will depend on the individual woman (Box 6.7). The main prophylactic strategies for menstrual migraine are listed in Tables 6.1 and 6.2.

Perimenstrual non-steroidal anti-inflammatory drugs

By inhibiting prostaglandin, trials show efficacy, particularly if accompanied by dysmenorrhoea and/or menorrhagia. ET com-

---

Box 6.7 **Perimenstrual versus continuous strategies for menstrual migraine**

Consider perimenstrual strategies for women with:
- predictable menstrual migraine
- regular menstrual cycles or use fertility monitor to predict menstruation
- no requirement for hormonal contraception
- debilitating, severe migraine pain which may recur or be of long duration

Consider continuous strategies for women with:
- additional migraine outside the perimenstrual phase
- irregular or unpredictable menstruation
- migraines unresponsive to perimenstrual prevention strategies
- requirement for hormonal contraception

---

menced perimenstrual mefenamic acid 500 mg tds two days prior to anticipated onset of menses and continued until the third day of bleeding.

Continuous hormonal prophylaxis

If hormonal contraception is required, menstrual migraine without aura may be improved by using continuous combined hormonal contraceptives or progestogen-only methods, which suppress ovulation and cause amenorrhoea. A risk versus benefit consideration is necessary for each woman. ET did not require a contraceptive strategy as her husband has had a vasectomy.

Perimenstrual oestrogen supplements

Only consider for women with regular and predictable menstruation. If other strategies fail, ET may try oestrogen supplementation when oestrogen is naturally declining before the onset of menses (Figure 6.6). No additional progestogens are necessary for endometrial protection provided a woman is producing her own natural progesterone. This can be checked by confirming ovulation with blood levels of progesterone seven days prior to anticipated menstruation. The level should be above 30 nmol/L. A home-use fertility monitor may be useful in both confirming ovulation and predicting menstruation. In women producing endogenous oestrogen, risk of cancer or thrombosis does not appear to increase.

This is hormonal supplementation rather than hormonal replacement therapy, which should only be considered if menopausal symptoms are evident. In both cases migraine is more likely to improve with the delivery of adequate, stable levels of oestrogen, i.e. by the transdermal route.

Outcome

Increasing sumatriptan to 100 mg resulted in less time lost from work, but relapse of symptoms over several days meant that ET was keen to find an effective preventive strategy. Perimenstrual mefenamic acid prevents ET's menstrual migraine attacks in most cycles and when they occur they are milder, with acute treatment working well. Her dysmenorrhoea and menorrhagia have improved. ET is aware that migraine may worsen during perimenopause but

Table 6.1 Perimenstrual prophylactic strategies for menstrual migraine

Strategy*	Who	Dose	Regimen	Main Side-Effects**	Main Contraindications**	Note
Mefenamic acid	Menstrual attacks on days 1–3 of bleeding Migraine associated with menorrhagia and/or dysmenorrhoea	500 mg 3–4 times daily	2–3 days before expected onset of menstruation until first 2–3 days of bleeding	Gastrointestinal disturbances and bleeding	Peptic ulcer and aspirin-induced allergy	Can start on day 1 of bleeding if menstruation irregular. Can be used for duration of bleeding. Also helps menorrhagia and dysmenorrhoea
Naproxen	Menstrual attacks on days 1–3 of bleeding Migraine associated with dysmenorrhoea	550 mg 1–2 times daily	5–7 days before expected onset of menstruation until day 5–7 of cycle	"	"	Alternative to mefenamic acid but less effective for menorrhagia
Perimenstrual estradiol gel/patches	Regular and predictable menses Must be ovulating (check progesterone level)	1.5 mg in 2.5 g gel; 100 µg patch	Three days before expected onset of menstruation for seven days total	Breast tenderness, fluid retention, nausea and leg cramps due to excess oestrogen	Risk of pregnancy, undiagnosed vaginal bleeding, oestrogen-dependent tumours, history of venous thromboembolism	Percutaneous provides higher, more stable levels of oestrogen than oral formulations. Reduce to 50 µg patch if effective but not well tolerated. If attacks delayed rather than aborted, continue until day 7 of cycle with tapered dose reduction over last two days
Frovatriptan	Regular and predictable menses	5 mg twice daily on first day of treatment; 2.5 mg twice daily on days 2–6 of treatment	Two days before expected onset of menstrual migraine for six days total	Flushing, tingling, drowsiness, dizziness, weakness, feeling of warmth or coldness, tightness in throat or chest	Uncontrolled hypertension, family history of coronary artery disease or heart attack, history of stroke, risk factors for coronary artery disease, uncontrolled diabetes	Perimenstrual prophylaxis with triptans limits their use for acute treatment
Naratriptan	Regular and predictable menses	1 mg twice daily	Three days before expected onset of menstrual migraine for six days total	"	"	"
Zolmitriptan	Regular and predictable menses	2.5 mg two or three times a day	Two days before expected onset of menstruation for seven days total	"	"	"
Sumatriptan	Regular and predictable menses	25 mg three times daily	Two to three days before expected onset of menstrual migraine for five days total	"	"	"

*These strategies are not licensed for the prophylaxis of menstrual migraine and clinical trial evidence showing efficacy is limited.
**Consult drug formulary for full details.

Table 6.2 Continuous hormonal prophylactic strategies for menstrual migraine

Strategy*	Example	Who	Regimen	Inhibit ovulation?	Main Side-effects**	Main Contraindications**	Note
Continuous combined hormonal contraceptives	Off-licence prescription of currently available 21/7 contraceptives (Lybrel® is a 365-day pill but not currently available in the UK)	Migraine in hormone-free week, Contraception required, Irregular/unpredictable menses, Easy reversibility preferred	Tricycle (three consecutive packs before a break) or continuous use without hormone-free interval	Yes	Nausea, oedema, breakthrough bleeding	Should not be used by women with migraine with aura because of increased stroke risk	Follow standard prescribing guidelines for contraindications
Progestogen only by intramuscular route or Subdermal route	Medroxyprogesterone acetate (Depo-Provera®), Etonorgestrel (Implanon®)	Contraception required, Irregular/unpredictable menses	Every three months, Three years	Yes	Irregular bleeding in early months often associated with headache, which usually improves when amenorrhoeic	Risk factors/known cardiovascular disease, breast cancer, hepatic disease, undiagnosed vaginal bleeding, suspected pregnancy	Follow standard prescribing recommendations
Progestogen only by intrauterine route	Levonorgestrel (Mirena®) Intrauterine System	Migraine associated with menorrhagia and/or dysmenorrhoea	Five years	No	"	"	Not effective against oestrogen withdrawal as migraine trigger
Progestogen only by oral route	Desogestrel (Cerazette®)	Irregular/unpredictable menses	Daily pill	Yes	"	"	Standard contraceptive oral progestogens are ineffective
Gonadotrophin-releasing hormone analogues	Goserelin acetate (Zoladex®)	Severe, refractory menstrual migraine, Other menstrual problems, Failure of other strategies	Every 28 days	Yes	Oestrogen deficiency including hot flushes, bone loss, vaginal dryness	Pregnancy, breastfeeding, undiagnosed vaginal bleeding	Requires regular monitoring in specialist department. Continuous oestrogen and progestogen 'add-back' therapy can be given to counter side-effects

*These strategies are not licensed for the prophylaxis of menstrual migraine and clinical trial evidence showing efficacy is limited.

**Consult drug formulary for full details.

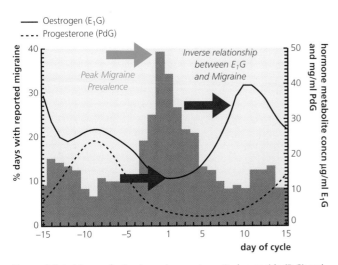

Figure 6.6 Incidence of migraine, urinary estrone-3-glucuronide (E$_1$G) and pregnanediol-3-glucuronide (PdG) levels on each day of the menstrual cycle in 120 cycles from 38 women
Source: MacGregor EA, Frith A, Ellis J, Aspinall L, Hackshaw A. Incidence of migraine relative to menstrual cycle phases of rising and falling estrogen. *Neurology* 2006; **67**: 2154–8.

that it is likely to improve post-menopause. She feels confident to be in control of her headaches once again.

Further reading

Loder E, Rizzoli P, Golub J. Hormonal management of migraine associated with menses and the menopause: a clinical review. *Headache* 2007; **47**: 329–40.

MacGregor EA. Menstrual migraine: a clinical review. *J Fam Plann Reprod Healthcare* 2007; **33(1)**: 36–47.

MacGregor EA, Frith A, Ellis J, Aspinall L. Predicting menstrual migraine with a home-use fertility monitor. *Neurology* 2005; **64**: 561–3.

MacGregor EA, Frith A, Ellis J, Aspinall L, Hackshaw A. Incidence of migraine relative to menstrual cycle phases of rising and falling estrogen. *Neurology* 2006; **67**: 2154–8.

Martin VT, Behbehani M. Ovarian hormones and migraine headache: understanding mechanisms and pathogenesis – Part 1. *Headache* 2006; **46**: 3–23.

Steiner TJ, MacGregor EA, Davies PTG. *Guidelines for All Healthcare Professionals in the Diagnosis and Management of Migraine, Tension-Type, Cluster and Medication Overuse Headache* (3rd edition 2007): www.bash.org.uk

CHAPTER 7

Childhood Periodic Syndromes

Ishaq Abu-Arafeh

OVERVIEW

- Abdominal migraine, cyclical vomiting syndrome, benign paroxysmal vertigo and benign paroxysmal torticollis of infancy are closely related to migraine

- The diagnosis of each disorder is based on well-defined clinical criteria and the absence of abnormalities on clinical examination

- The treatment of childhood syndromes related to migraine should be as simple as possible

- Drug prophylaxis is necessary only for a small number of children with abdominal migraine and cyclical vomiting syndrome

- Children with these conditions can continue to suffer as adults; migraine may be additional to or replace the related disorder

- The incidence of migraine is greater than expected among first-degree relatives of these children

CASE HISTORY 1

The girl with recurrent episodic vomiting
Jenny first presented at the age of 18 months with recurrent episodes of being unwell, looking pale, crying in pain and vomiting. During the episodes she held her head tilted to one side. There was no fever, rash, respiratory symptoms or loss of consciousness. She recovered after two or three days and returned to her normal self. The episodes occurred once every 2–3 months. Around the age of three years, the episodes became prolonged, with intense nausea, vomiting, lethargy and pallor and occasionally required hospital admission for treatment of dehydration. She had no apparent head tilt. All investigations, including metabolic, microbiological and appropriate imaging, showed no identifiable underlying cause. By the age of six years, she started to complain of throbbing and unilateral headache during the episodes, in addition to her usual symptoms. Physical examination continued to be normal throughout this time.

CASE HISTORY 2

The boy with recurrent episodic abdominal pain
Ali is a seven-year-old boy who presented to his general practitioner with episodes of abdominal pain. His mother described him crying in pain, looking pale, refusing to eat and complaining of nausea. He would also point to the centre of his abdomen around the umbilicus. His mother is concerned because the episodes are occurring at least once a month and last for up to 24 hours; he has vomited on several occasions. Between attacks Ali is well and enjoys school.

His mother suffers from migraine; his younger brother and his father are both well and healthy.

Physical examination shows no abnormalities. His weight and height are on the 75th percentile and his blood count, serum electrolytes, blood glucose and liver function tests are normal.

History

Important features to elicit in the history are the duration of illness, the frequency and duration of each attack, and the severity of symptoms or pain. The history should include a full description of the associated symptoms of each disorder, including the presence or absence of anorexia, nausea, vomiting and other sensory, motor or autonomic symptoms. The child may be able to identify relieving factors such as rest, sleep and medication. Full medication history should be taken to include the doses, format, time of administration and frequency of the use of rescue treatment, as well as the doses and length of course of preventive treatment.

Examination

Full physical and neurological assessment during and between attacks is essential. A normal examination during and between attacks is important in order to exclude gastrointestinal, renal or metabolic disorders, as well as an underlying brain disorder. Assessment may need to be repeated on more than one occasion to confirm the normal findings. Physical examination should include

ABC of Headache. Edited by A. MacGregor & A. Frith.
© 2009 Blackwell Publishing, ISBN 978-1-4051-7066-6.

Box 7.1 **Minimum investigations of a child with recurrent episodic vomiting or abdominal pain**

- Urine culture
- Blood count and biochemical screen, including acute phase reactants such as C-reactive protein and erythrocyte sedimentation rate
- Abdominal ultrasound during an attack, looking particularly for renal enlargement
- Urine examination for amino acids, short chain organic acids and porphyrins during an attack; ketones are normally present in the urine during an attack of CVS, giving rise to acidosis as an alternative name for the syndrome
- Acid–base balance, lactate/pyruvate ratio and ammonia during an attack

measuring the blood pressure, and neurological examination should include measuring head circumference, ophthalmoscopy and cerebellar function assessment.

Examination should include measurement of weight and height to confirm normal growth and absence of malabsorption syndromes.

Investigations

Investigations to consider in cases of recurrent episodic attacks of vomiting or abdominal pain are shown in Box 7.1.

It is necessary to exclude a posterior fossa brain tumour by brain imaging (CT or MRI scan) if there are any concerning symptoms or signs in the history and examination. Neuroimaging is mandatory if symptoms and signs suggestive of cerebellar dysfunction, such as nystagmus, ataxia and hand incoordination, are present.

Prospective diaries of episodes may also be helpful in confirming frequency and duration of attacks and also in identifying other subtle associated symptoms that may be helpful in suspecting or excluding other disorders.

Diagnosis

Differential diagnosis

It is appropriate to look at all symptoms that start in early childhood as a continuum probably related to one disorder before exploring the possibility of different diseases.

Benign paroxysmal torticollis of infancy (BPTI), cyclical vomiting syndrome (CVS), abdominal migraine and benign paroxysmal vertigo (BPV) are common childhood syndromes that share epidemiological and clinical features with migraine. The four conditions have been shown to coexist in the same patient or the same family. Patients may suffer from CVS, BPTI or abdominal migraine and develop typical childhood migraine headache in late childhood or early adult life. The conditions share clinical features of well-defined attacks with complete return to normality in between. The shared clinical features include pain, vasomotor symptoms (mainly pallor), gastrointestinal manifestations such as anorexia, nausea and vomiting, and sensory disturbances such as light and noise intolerance. BPTI and migraine share genetic predisposition on

Box 7.2 **International Classification of Headache Disorders. Diagnostic criteria for benign paroxysmal torticollis of infancy**

Diagnostic criteria
A. Episodic attacks, in a young child, with all of the following characteristics and fulfilling criterion B:
  1. tilt of the head to one side (not always the same side), with or without slight rotation
  2. lasting minutes to days
  3. remitting spontaneously and tending to recur monthly
B. During attacks, symptoms and/or signs of one or more of the following:
  1. pallor
  2. irritability
  3. malaise
  4. vomiting
  5. ataxia
C. Normal neurological examination between attacks
D. Not attributed to another disorder

Source: Headache Classification Subcommittee of the International Headache Society (IHS). *The International Classification of Headache Disorders* (2nd edition). *Cephalalgia* 2004; **24** (suppl 1): 1–160.

Box 7.3 **International Classification of Headache Disorders. Diagnostic criteria for benign paroxysmal vertigo of childhood**

Diagnostic criteria
A. At least five attacks fulfilling criterion B
B. Multiple episodes of severe vertigo,[1] occurring without warning and resolving spontaneously after minutes to hours
C. Normal neurological examination, audiometric and vestibular functions between attacks
D. Normal electroencephalogram

Note:
1. Often associated with nystagmus or vomiting; unilateral throbbing headache may occur in some attacks.
Source: Headache Classification Subcommittee of the International Headache Society (IHS). *The International Classification of Headache Disorders* (2nd edition). *Cephalalgia* 2004; **24** (suppl 1): 1–160.

CACNA1A (the calcium channel gene), suggesting ion channel disorder as a likely underlying pathogenesis. Migraine, CVS and abdominal migraine have a strong familial predisposition and share common responses to medical treatment.

The diagnosis of BPTI is based on the clinical presentation of discrete episodes of head tilt with return to normality between attacks (Box 7.2). BPV can be excluded because there is no vertigo or nystagmus (Box 7.3). Other conditions to be excluded (Box 7.4) include Gradenigo's syndrome, an inflammatory, commonly infectious, process in the cerebello-pontine area secondary to chronic or recurrent otitis media. In this condition, torticollis is typically associated with a history of ear infections, fever, headache and abducens palsy.

Box 7.4 **Differential diagnosis of BPTI**

- Focal idiopathic or dystonia secondary to structural, metabolic or toxic disorders of the CNS
- Dystonic cerebral palsy
- Extrapyramidal side-effects of medications such as metoclopramide
- Posterior fossa brain tumour
- Gradenigo's syndrome

Box 7.5 **International Classification of Headache Disorders. Diagnostic criteria for cyclical vomiting**

Diagnostic criteria
A. At least five attacks fulfilling criteria B and C
B. Episodic attacks, stereotypical in the individual patient, of intense nausea and vomiting lasting from one hour to five days
C. Vomiting during attacks occurs at least four times an hour for at least one hour
D. Symptom-free between attacks
E. Not attributed to any other disorder

Source: Headache Classification Subcommittee of the International Headache Society (IHS). *The International Classification of Headache Disorders* (2nd edition). *Cephalalgia* 2004; **24** (suppl 1): 1–160.

Box 7.6 **Differential diagnosis of CVS**

- Food intolerance
- Coeliac disease
- Inflammatory bowel disease
- Metabolic disorders
- Infection, e.g. recurrent urinary tract infection or otitis media
- Renal tract obstruction
- Raised intracranial pressure

Box 7.7 **International Classification of Headache Disorders. Diagnostic criteria for abdominal migraine**

Diagnostic criteria
A. At least five attacks fulfilling criteria B–D
B. Attacks of abdominal pain lasting 1–72 hours (untreated or unsuccessfully treated)
C. Abdominal pain has all of the following characteristics:
    1. midline location, periumbilical or poorly localized
    2. dull or 'just sore' quality
    3. moderate or severe intensity
D. During abdominal pain at least two of the following:
    1. anorexia
    2. nausea
    3. vomiting
    4. pallor
E. Not attributed to another disorder

Source: Headache Classification Subcommittee of the International Headache Society (IHS). *The International Classification of Headache Disorders* (2nd edition). *Cephalalgia* 2004; **24** (suppl 1): 1–160.

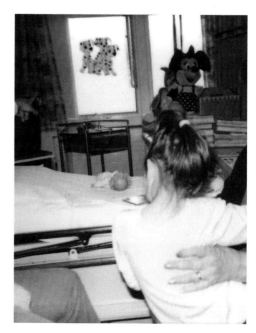

Figure 7.1 Head tilt to the right during an episode of BPTI

The presentation of Jenny, the girl with recurrent episodes of vomiting (case 1), is suggestive of CVS. As with BPTI, diagnosis of CVS is based on taking a good history of the attacks and establishing complete return to normality between attacks (Box 7.5). The differential diagnosis includes inter-current illnesses, viral infections, food intolerance and other chronic diseases of the gastrointestinal tract (Box 7.6).

The most likely diagnosis for Ali (case 2), based on the symptoms and the normal examination, is abdominal migraine (Box 7.7). In the absence of a diagnostic test, the diagnosis is one of exclusion. There is neither diarrhoea nor constipation in abdominal migraine, a feature that distinguishes it from irritable bowel syndrome.

Final diagnosis

Case 1

Jenny's initial symptoms of unexplained episodes of head tilt alarmed her parents, although she had no other symptoms and continued being well throughout the episode, which lasted 2–3 days (Figure 7.1). The recurrence of the episodes over a period of two years, absence of possible causes of dystonia, such as the use of anti-emetic medications, and the lack of abnormal findings on physical and neurological examination during and between attacks suggested a diagnosis of BPTI. As BPTI resolved over a period of 2–3 years, Jenny started to suffer from unexplained and regularly relapsing episodes of intense nausea and vomiting. The features of these episodes as described above are consistent with CVS (Figures 7.2–7.4).

By the age of 5–6 years, the episodes of CVS showed further transformation to indicate the presence of severe throbbing headache typical of migraine without aura.

It is unusual to see all three disorders in one child with such a graphic transformation, but this case demonstrates the different

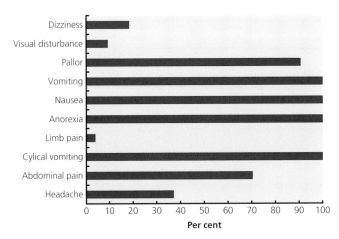

Figure 7.2 Symptom spectrum in 54 children with cyclical vomiting
Source: Clinic data (courtesy of George Russell, Aberdeen).

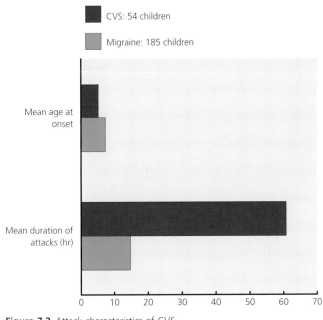

Figure 7.3 Attack characteristics of CVS
Source: Clinic data (courtesy of George Russell, Aberdeen).

syndromes related to migraine and is a good reminder of the possible common clinical and pathological underlying mechanisms.

Case 2

Abdominal migraine is a common disorder affecting around 4% of schoolchildren with variable severity and frequency of attacks. It affects younger age groups with mean age of onset of eight years. Many children have coexisting migraine headache, family history of migraine or grow up to have migraine as adults.

Management

Management of BPTI

On making the diagnosis the parents are reassured about the benign course of the condition and of the complete recovery over a period of 2–3 years. No specific treatment is required or effective.

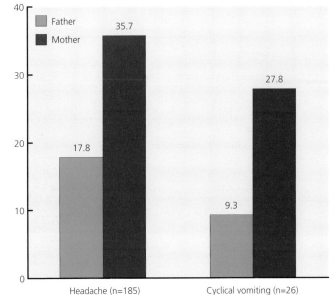

Figure 7.4 Family history of migraine in children with CVS
Source: Dignan F, Symon DNK, Abu-Arafeh I, Russell G. The prognosis of cyclical vomiting syndrome. *Arch Dis Child* 2001; **84**: 55–7.

Management of CVS

Management of acute episodes should be started as early as possible after the onset of symptoms and before the start of vomiting. Initial symptoms of pallor, lethargy and nausea should alert the child and parents to the need for early treatment. Children are given the chance to lie down and rest, given small and frequent amounts of fluids and, at an early stage, are given anti-emetic medications. Oral ondansetron has proved effective in the melt formula. If oral medications become intolerable, other routes for administering medications may be necessary. Prevention of dehydration is an important objective. If oral fluid replacement is unsuccessful, admission to hospital for intravenous treatment is an appropriate option. Each child with CVS should have a care plan agreed by parents, general practitioner and hospital paediatrician for the management of acute attacks.

Preventive treatment, including pizotifen, amitriptyline or erythromycin, may be necessary in children with frequent episodes requiring hospital admissions. Encouraging a healthy lifestyle with regular meals, regular sleep and regular exercise can help reduce the frequency of attacks.

Management of abdominal migraine

The aim of management of abdominal migraine is to make a full assessment of the child, exclude other treatable organic causes of recurrent abdominal pain and gain the confidence of the child and the parents that their concerns are being taken seriously and are properly addressed.

On occasions, explanation and reassurance may be the only treatment needed. Such explanation should be followed by a thorough search for avoidable trigger factors, such as stress, travel, prolonged fasting, irregular sleeping habits, exposure to glaring or flickering lights, and exercise (Figure 7.5).

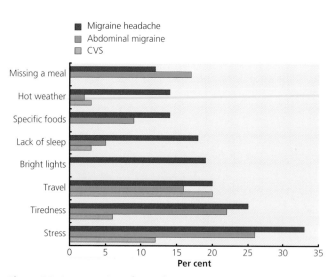

Figure 7.5 Common trigger factors for migraine, abdominal migraine and CVS
Source: Abu-Arafeh I. Russell G. Prevalence and clinical features of abdominal migraine compared with those of migraine headache. *Arch Dis Child* 1995; **72(5)**: 413–17.

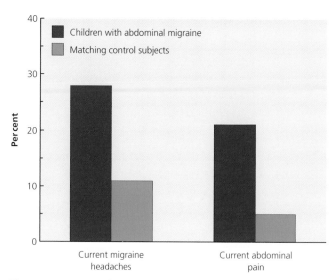

Figure 7.7 Prognosis of abdominal migraine after a mean of 10 years of diagnosis versus controls
Source: Dignan F, Abu-Arafeh I, Russell G. The prognosis of childhood abdominal migraine. *Arch Dis Child* 2001; **84**: 415–18.

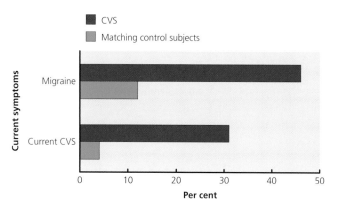

Figure 7.6 Prognosis of CVS after a mean of 10 years of diagnosis as compared to controls
Source: Dignan F, Symon DNK, Abu-Arafeh I, Russell G. The prognosis of cyclical vomiting syndrome. *Arch Dis Child* 2001; **84**: 5–7.

Rest and sleep are usually helpful in reducing the intensity of attack. Drug therapy for acute attacks is often precluded by anorexia, nausea and/or vomiting, but simple oral analgesics with or without metoclopramide or domperidone can be tried. The total dose given should be monitored to avoid toxic effects from sudden absorption at the end of the attack. Analgesic and/or anti-emetic suppositories are also useful.

Dietary management may be an alternative non-drug strategy, but with limited success, and may include the avoidance of foods rich in amines or xanthines, together with any foods that the family suspect are triggering attacks.

Drug prophylaxis has a limited part to play in the management of abdominal migraine. It is restricted to children who have not responded to non-drug measures and whose symptoms impact adversely on their lives. There is limited support for the use of pizotifen in a small double-blind, placebo-controlled trial, but other drugs, such as propranolol and cyproheptidine, may also be used.

Outcome

Childhood periodic symptoms are very much a disorder of early childhood with peak age of onset of 18 months for BPTI, 2–3 years for BPV, five years for CVS and 10 years for abdominal migraine. BPTI resolves completely by the age of three years and BPV resolves by age of five years. CVS and abdominal migraine may persist into adult life and around half the patients suffer from migraine headaches during late childhood and as adults (Figures 7.6 and 7.7).

Further reading

Abu-Arafeh I, Russell G. Prevalence and clinical features of abdominal migraine compared with those of migraine headache. *Arch Dis Child* 1995; **72**: 413–17.

Dignan F, Abu-Arafeh I, Russell G. The prognosis of childhood abdominal migraine. *Arch Dis Child* 2001; **84**: 415–18.

Dignan F, Symon DNK, Abu-Arafeh I, Russell G. The prognosis of cyclical vomiting syndrome. *Arch Dis Child* 2001; **84**: 55–7.

Russell G, Abu-Arafeh I. Childhood syndromes related to migraine. In *Childhood Headache, Clinics in Developmental Medicine*. Ed I Abu-Arafeh. London: MacKeith Press, 2002: 66–95.

Symon DN, Russell G. Double-blind placebo-controlled trial of pizotifen syrup in the treatment of abdominal migraine. *Arch Dis Child* 1995; **72**: 48–50.

CHAPTER 8

Teenage Headache

Ishaq Abu-Arafeh

OVERVIEW

- Headache is common in teenagers
- Migraine and tension-type headache are the most common causes
- Mixed headaches can confuse diagnosis and treatment
- Headache diaries are useful in making the diagnosis of different types of headache
- Emotional and psychological factors play an important role in daily headaches and should be considered in the assessment and management of teenagers with headache
- Headache can have a significant impact on education and family life
- Investigations are rarely needed if the history is typical and examination normal
- Explanation of the diagnosis and education of the teenager and the family improve compliance with advice and treatment
- Treatment should be individualized to the headache profile

CASE HISTORY

The girl with two different headaches

Amy, a 14-year-old, attends the clinic complaining of headache. Amy and her mother are concerned about the headaches as she is losing time from school. Amy lives with her mother and younger sister (11 years). Her parents separated two years ago and she and her sister spend one weekend every fortnight with their father and his partner.

History

How many different headache types does the patient have?

Amy describes two types of headache. Type 1 is 'bad'. Most are associated with anorexia, nausea, photophobia, phonophobia and pallor, but less than half the attacks are associated with vomiting. Type 2 is 'not so bad'. There is no nausea or vomiting and no intolerance to light or noise. In particular, she is able to have normal meals.

ABC of Headache. Edited by A. MacGregor & A. Frith.
© 2009 Blackwell Publishing, ISBN 978-1-4051-7066-6.

Time questions

Amy has had headaches for the past three years. She gets one or two type 1 headaches each month. The headache builds up in intensity over a period of 60 minutes and each attack lasts 12–24 hours. Type 2 headaches occur almost every day of the week and each attack lasts 2–3 hours.

Character questions

In type 1 the pain is throbbing in nature with maximum intensity around the forehead and one side of the head. Amy describes type 2 headaches as 'just sore' round the head.

Cause questions

There are no known warning symptoms or trigger factors.

Response to headache questions

With type 1 headaches Amy is unable to carry out any activities and is forced to lie down. She feels better after rest and sleep. Paracetamol helps a little, but she finds codeine more helpful in relieving symptoms.

Type 2 headaches are relieved with rest, but Amy only occasionally treats these headaches with paracetamol. These headaches affect her ability to concentrate on her schoolwork and she often stays at home.

State of health between attacks

Other than headaches, she is well and has no other illnesses.

Examination

Blood pressure and funduscopy are mandatory in any person presenting with headache. Head circumference should also be considered. In Amy's case physical and neurological examinations were normal. However, consider repeating the examination at a later date to confirm this.

As well as excluding serious underlying disorders such as a brain tumour, detailed assessment gives the teenager and parents the confidence that the doctor has taken their complaints seriously.

Investigations

CT or MRI scan is not usually necessary unless there are features suggestive of underlying organic disease (Box 8.1). A lower threshold for neuroimaging may be considered if there is any doubt about the physical findings or if there are inconsistent or fluctuating symptoms.

Measurement of CSF opening pressure is only rarely needed, but is necessary for the diagnosis of idiopathic intracranial hypertension in the presence of visual field impairment, papilloedema and normal MRI scan.

Diagnosis

Differential diagnosis

Amy presented with a chronic headache (three years' duration) occurring almost daily. The priority for the attending physician is to exclude at an early opportunity the possibility of an organic cause. An initial umbrella diagnosis of chronic daily headache is considered at the early assessment (Figure 8.1).

The normal health, the absence of other symptoms indicating raised intracranial pressure or cerebellar dysfunction, the complete resolution of symptoms between attacks and the normal physical and neurological examination make it extremely unlikely that this child has a brain tumour as the underlying cause of her headaches.

The intermittent nature of the headache attacks, the absence of visual field defects and newly presenting squint (VI nerve palsy), the absence of papilloedema and risk factors make the diagnosis of idiopathic intracranial hypertension very unlikely.

Full symptom analysis and diary recording help to identify the nature of different headache attacks on different days over a period of time (Box 8.2).

Migraine is the most likely diagnosis of the type 1 headaches (Box 8.3) and affects around 1 in 10 schoolchildren and 1 in 5 teenage girls (Figure 8.2).

Box 8.1 Indications for neuroimaging in children with chronic headache

- Features of cerebellar dysfunction
    - ataxia
    - nystagmus
    - intention tremor
- Features of increased intracranial pressure
    - papilloedema
    - night or early morning vomiting
    - large head
- New focal neurological deficits including recent squint
- Seizures, especially focal
- Personality change
- Unexplained deterioration of schoolwork

Box 8.2 Diary

Name: Date of birth: Sex:
Address:

Attack number	1	2	3	4	5
Date					
Time started					
Time resolved					
Severity of headache*					
Type of headache**					
What may have started it?					
Any loss of appetite?					
Nausea?					
Vomiting?					
Does light make it worse?					
Does noise make it worse?					
Is it made worse by walking?					
Does rest make it better?					
Does sleep make it better?					
Is it better after paracetamol?					

*Severity: Write 1 if headache is not interfering with normal activities
                    Write 2 if headache is interfering with some activities
                    Write 3 if headache is interfering with all activities
**Type of pain: Choose one of the following or your own descriptions:
                    Throbbing, hitting, banging, tightness, pressure, squeezing, sharp, stabbing, dull or can't describe

---

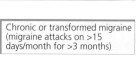

Figure 8.1 Differential diagnosis of a teenager with chronic daily headache

Brain tumour (signs of raised intracranial pressure)

Hydrocephalus (large head, VP shunt)

Idiopathic intracranial hypertension (papilloedema, squint, CSF pressure >250 mm H_2O)

A teenager with chronic daily headache

Analgesia overuse headache (painkillers taken >2 days/week for >3 months)

Chronic tension type headache (tension headaches on >15 days/month for >3 months)

Chronic or transformed migraine (migraine attacks on >15 days/month for >3 months)

Mixed types of headache

Box 8.3 **International Classification of Headache Disorders. Diagnostic criteria for migraine without aura**

Diagnostic criteria
A. At least five attacks fulfilling criteria B–D
B. Headache lasting 1–72 hours (untreated or unsuccessfully treated)
C. Headache has at least two of the following characteristics:
    1. unilateral location (frontal and bi-temporal locations are common in children)
    2. pulsating quality
    3. moderate or severe intensity (inhibits or prohibits daily activities)
    4. aggravated by walking upstairs or similar routine physical activity
D. During headache, at least one of the following:
    1. nausea and/or vomiting
    2. photophobia or phonophobia (symptoms can be inferred from behaviour)
E. No evidence of organic disease

Source: adapted from Headache Classification Subcommittee of the International Headache Society (IHS), *The International Classification of Headache Disorders* (2nd edition). *Cephalalgia* 2004; **24** (suppl 1): 1–160.

Box 8.4 **International Classification of Headache Disorders. Diagnostic criteria for tension-type headache**

	Infrequent	Frequent	Chronic
Diagnostic criteria			
A. Frequency:	<12 days/year	12–180 days/year	>180 days/year
B. Duration:	30 minutes– 7 days		hours– continuous

C. At least three of the following;
    1. pressing/tightening quality
    2. mild to moderate severity
    3. bilateral location
    4. not aggravated by walking
D. Both of the following;
    1. no nausea (anorexia may occur)
    2. no photophobia or phonophobia
E. Not attributed to any other disorder

Source: adapted from Headache Classification Subcommittee of the International Headache Society (IHS), *The International Classification of Headache Disorders* (2nd edition). *Cephalalgia* 2004; **24** (suppl 1): 1–160.

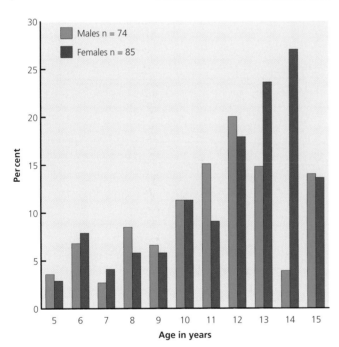

Figure 8.2 Prevalence of migraine among children
Source: adapted from Abu-Arefeh I, Russell G. Prevalence of headache and migraine in schoolchildren. *BMJ* 1994; **309**: 765–9.

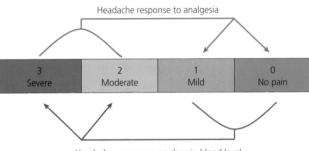

Figure 8.3 Analgesic overuse headache: the aim of treatment is to alleviate pain (severe or moderate pain to mild or absent), but analgesia overuse may lead to frequent recurrence of headache

1%. Changing frequency of headache attacks over a long period of time may identify the transformation of episodic tension-type headache into chronic tension headache. However, in some children chronic tension-type headache may start from the early presentation as newly presenting chronic daily headache.

Medication overuse headache should be considered if painkillers are taken on at least 15 days a month over a period of at least three months (Figure 8.3). There is no evidence that Amy is taking excessive amounts of analgesics as she does not treat the daily tension headaches, except occasionally with paracetamol.

Preliminary diagnosis

Prospective headache diaries can confirm the clinical features of each different type of headache. The likely diagnosis is episodic migraine without aura and chronic tension-type headache.

Initial management

Children with chronic daily headache, commonly due to tension headache, are more likely to seek medical advice than children with episodic headache and may be disproportionately represented in

Since Amy has discrete attacks no more than twice a month, chronic migraine or transformed migraine is unlikely to be the cause of the daily headaches. In chronic migraine, attacks of headache fulfilling the criteria for the diagnosis of migraine occur on a daily or almost daily basis.

Type 2 headaches are typical of tension-type headache (Box 8.4). Infrequent and frequent tension-type headache affect 12–25% of children; prevalence of chronic tension-type headache is less than

Box 8.5 Common reasons for children with headache seeking medical advice

- Parents' misconception that teenagers should not have headache
- Concerns regarding sinister cause (brain tumour)
- Headache has been going on for a long time
- Missing too many schooldays because of headache
- Headache affecting schoolwork
- Uncertain diagnosis
- Poor response to medications
- Overuse of medication

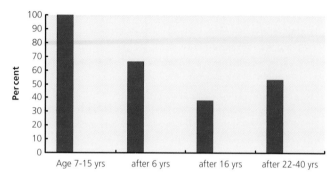

Figure 8.4 Prognosis of childhood migraine over 40 years' follow-up: a study of 73 schoolchildren
Source: adapted from Bille B. A 40-year follow-up of school children with migraine. *Cephalalgia* 1997; **17**: 488–91.

Table 8.1 Medications used in the acute treatment of migraine attacks

Drug	Age	
	Under 12 years*	**12–18 years**
Paracetamol		
Dose	10–20 mg/kg	500–1000 mg
Maximum no. of doses/24 hr	4	4
Maximum total dose/24 hr	100 mg/kg	8000 mg
Ibuprofen		
Dose	10–15 mg/kg	400 mg
Maximum no. of doses/24 hr	4	4
Maximum total dose/24 hr	60 mg/kg	1600 mg
Metoclopramide		
Dose	100 mcg/kg	2.5–10 mg
Maximum no. of doses/24 hr	3	4
Maximum total dose/24 hr	300 mcg/kg	40 mg
Domperidone		
Dose	0.25–0.5 mg/kg	10–20 mg
Maximum no. of doses/24 hr	4	4
Maximum total dose/24 hr	2.4 mg/kg	80 mg
Sumatriptan (intranasal only)		
Dose	Not indicated	10 mg
Maximum no. of doses/24 hr		2
Maximum total dose/24 hr		20 mg
Diclofenac	6 months–18 years	
Dose	0.3–1.0 mg/kg	
Maximum no. of doses/24 hr	3	
Maximum total dose/24 hr	150 mg	

*Maximum doses in under 12 s should never exceed the 12–18 years doses

paediatric neurology and specialist headache clinics, accounting for up to one-third of the patients with headache.

Understanding the reasons for specialist referral is important in order to reassure the family and to address their concerns (Box 8.5). Assessing the impact of the headache on Amy and the rest of her family is an integral part of management. Chronic headache may interfere with school attendance and education, and this will cause anxiety to the parents and stress to the teenager. Frequent or unpredictable headache may cause disruption to normal family social life and recreation activities, limiting family outings, interaction and leisure time. Addressing these issues should be direct and supportive and may be delivered in the clinic or by an experienced clinical psychologist.

Educating Amy and her parents on the natural course of headache will help in achieving better understanding of symptoms and appropriate use of, and adherence to, treatment. Frequency of migraine fluctuates considerably over time (Figure 8.4).

Amy should be encouraged to identify and avoid headache trigger factors if at all possible. A healthy lifestyle may help to reduce frequency of attacks by avoiding erratic meal and sleep patterns, avoiding excessive intake of analgesia and taking regular exercise.

Managing migraine
Symptomatic treatment
Amy should treat migraine attacks as soon as possible after the onset of headache and before the headache becomes severe or

associated with nausea and vomiting. For effective pain relief analgesics should be given in optimum doses (Table 8.1). If simple analgesics are given in adequate dosage, there is seldom any further benefit from using opiates such as codeine. Amy should be encouraged to lie down or sleep.

Oral administration is the preferred route of medications unless nausea and vomiting are early symptoms. In such cases, early treatment with an anti-emetic drug such as cyclizine, domperidone or metoclopramide may offer good relief of nausea and may improve the response to painkillers. Otherwise, nasal administration may offer a good alternative. Sumatriptan as a nasal spray (10 mg) is licensed for children over the age of 12 years and has been shown to be effective in many but not all patients.

Prophylactic treatment
Preventative treatment of migraine would be indicated if Amy had at least four occasions a month which were severe and long enough to stop activities, and simple lifestyle measures were ineffective. No prophylactic prevents every headache, but pizotifen, propranolol and possibly topiramate may offer some relief in frequency or severity (Table 8.2). Medication should be taken regularly for at least two months in appropriate dosages before their success or failure can be confidently decided.

Table 8.2 Medications used in the prevention of migraine attacks

Drug	Dose	
	Under 12 years*	**12–18 years**
Pizotifen	0.5–1.0 mg/day Single dose – night	1.5–3.0 mg/day Single dose – night
Propranolol	0.2–0.5 mg/kg Max. 4 mg/kg/day	2–3 mg/kg/day Max. 160 mg/day
Amitriptyline	not indicated for under 12 years	Up to 50 mg/night
Topiramate	not indicated for under 12 years	2–3 mg/kg/day
		Gradual increase to target dose

*Maximum doses in under 12s should not exceed the 12–18 years doses.

Managing tension-type headache

The management of episodic tension-type headache can be tailored to suit the individual. Simple analgesics are safe and effective and should be used early and in the full recommended dose. However, they should not be used more often than 2–3 days a week, otherwise chronic daily headache, as a result of medication overuse, is a real risk. In such cases, analgesia should be withdrawn in order to achieve resolution of the daily headache. The withdrawal of analgesia can cause apprehension and worry, and also a transient worsening of the headache. If children and parents are warned of possible worsening of symptoms during the first week of withdrawal, compliance with advice is usually good and improvement follows.

Managing Amy's chronic tension headache consists of reassurance regarding the benign nature of the disorder, encouraging her to adopt a healthy lifestyle if appropriate, such as taking regular meals, regular sleep and regular exercise and rest. Amy should be encouraged to review her intake of caffeine-containing drinks and reduce as much as possible or even stop them completely. In many children such simple measures may be enough to help them overcome the impact of daily headache without resorting to medications. However, by avoiding painkillers Amy may find the headaches

are unbearable and therefore a pain-modulating agent such as amitriptyline may help in reducing the headache.

If Amy's headache continues to be a problem, a clinical psychologist may be able to help Amy to understand her headache, devise coping strategies and may help her modify her responses to pain. Treatment may consist of cognitive behavioural therapy (CBT), biofeedback and/or relaxation techniques.

Final diagnosis

Migraine without aura and chronic tension-type headache.

Outcome

The natural course of migraine is one of remissions and relapses. Amy and her mother are told to expect good spells with a few or no headaches that may last for months or years and also bad spells with frequent headaches at times. In general, as children grow older, migraine headaches tend to become less frequent and in some people the attacks become so infrequent they feel that headache stopped completely (Figure 8.4). Tension headache behaves in similar manner and can recur, though the patient should expect good long periods of remissions.

Further reading

Abu-Arafeh I. Chronic tension-type headache in children and adolescents. *Cephalalgia* 2001; **21**: 830–6.

Abu-Arafeh I (Ed). *Childhood Headache, Clinics in Developmental Medicine*, Volume 158. London: MacKeith Press, 2002.

Bille B. A 40-year follow-up of school children with migraine. *Cephalalgia* 1997; **17**: 488–91.

Lewis D, Ashwal S, Hershey A, Hirtz D, Yonker M, Silberstein S. Practice parameter: pharmacological treatment of migraine headache in children and adolescents: report of the American Academy of Neurology Quality Standards Subcommittee and the Practice Committee of the Child Neurology Society. *Neurology* 2004; **63**: 2215–24.

Ryan S. Medicines for migraine, *Arch Dis Child Ed Pract* 2007; **92**: 50–5.

Seshia SS. Chronic daily headache in children and adolescents. *Can J Neurol Sci* 2004; **31**: 319–23.

CHAPTER 9

Exertional Headache

R. Allan Purdy

OVERVIEW

- Exertional headache is a common but under-recognised disorder
- The history is very important as there are no clinical signs
- Secondary causes have to be sought if the history indicates atypical features
- Referral is indicated if patients need further diagnostic considerations regarding investigation or treatment

CASE HISTORY

The woman with exercise headache

WD is 22. She has headaches worse with exercise. She can only run one or two lengths of the gymnasium without getting a headache; in the past she could at least run up to 4 km on occasion. Her headache was worse with coughing or sneezing as well as with other forms of exertion, such as walking upstairs. She has no nausea or vomiting, no visual disturbance or aura. Lights, sounds or smells do not affect the headache, and there are no food triggers. The headache is not localised in any particular place but she points to both temples, the vertex of the head and down the back of her head. Interestingly WD's headache has a lot of qualities including 'sharpness', sometimes like a 'headache' or like a 'pain', and other times it feels like there is a 'chisel' in her head. Sometimes there is 'thumping', but there are no jabs or jolts.

History

How many different headache types does the patient experience?

Although WD has many qualities to her headache and it occurs in many parts of her head, it sounds like one headache type that is made worse by exertion. If this is the case and there are no other clinical characteristics of concern then a primary cause is most likely.

Time questions

It is important to get more clinical information on the timing of her headaches. WD indicates that originally the headaches were

infrequent after the first one, but are now becoming more frequent. They have ranged in severity of 3–4/10 and in the background and can go up to 8–9/10 when severe. The 'bad' ones, again worse with exertion, can last several hours in duration.

Character questions

As indicated, the headache has different characteristics which is not unusual in headache patients and at this stage does not help with determining if the headaches are primary or secondary in nature.

Cause questions

WD has a significant important historical fact in her headache history that cannot be ignored and is important to know in order to direct her care and, if necessary, investigation and/or treatment. Her headache began after being on an amusement ride. It was a high-velocity, spinning ride, in which each passenger spins 360 degrees as an entire arm of the ride goes 360 degrees. On ending this ride, she experienced headache, which was only about 6/10.

Response to headache questions

WD has no prior history of headache and there is no family history of neurological disease, headache or migraine. She has been given various medications for her headaches without relief, including analgesics such as paracetamol or acetylsalicylic acid for acute pain and ketorolac, sodium valproate and flunarizine for headache prevention. Bilateral occipital nerve blocks with a local anaesthetic and steroid were tried as well as some massage therapy, both unhelpful.

State of health between attacks

WD has been healthy other than her headaches. She has no medical or surgical illnesses otherwise, is happily attending university without undue stress and she denied depression. She does not smoke or drink and had no allergies.

Examination

Blood pressure was 116/60; heart rate 72 and normal. The rest of her general and neurological examinations were normal.

Investigations

Initially having a moderately severe headache for the first time in her life, she went to a local hospital for some testing. She had CT

ABC of Headache. Edited by A. MacGregor & A. Frith.
© 2009 Blackwell Publishing, ISBN 978-1-4051-7066-6.

head scan and lumbar puncture (LP) and cerebrospinal fluid (CSF) examination, which were negative. Nothing further should have been considered at this stage.

Diagnosis

Differential diagnosis

In the absence of clinical signs, a primary headache is likely. Primary exertional headaches are described as aching, pounding, or pulsating (Box 9.1). They occur at the peak of exercise and subside with cessation. Primary exertional headache occurs in hot weather and at high altitude. Caffeine, poor nutrition, hypoglycemia, and

---

Box 9.1 **International Classification of Headache Disorders. Diagnostic criteria for primary exertional headache**

Previously used terms:
Benign exertional headache

Diagnostic criteria:
A. Pulsating headache fulfilling criteria B and C
B. Lasting from 5 minutes to 48 hours
C. Brought on by and occurring only during or after physical exertion
D. Not attributed to another disorder

Source: Headache Classification Subcommittee of the International Headache Society (IHS). *The International Classification of Headache Disorders* (2nd edition). *Cephalalgia* 2004; **24** (suppl 1): 1–160.

---

alcohol usage may be contributing factors. They can occur in poorly conditioned people who exercise infrequently and in trained athletes. They may have many characteristics of migraine with associated nausea, vomiting, and photophobia, and can be unilateral or bilateral. The aetiology of primary exertional headache is unknown but may be related to extracranial and intracranial cerebral vasodilatation. The prognosis for patients with primary headache is good. However, primary exertional headache must be a diagnosis of exclusion (Figure 9.1), as other primary headache disorders can also be worse with exertion or other activities. These include primary cough headache (Box 9.2), and primary headache associated with sexual activity (Box 9.3). Also it is important to understand that migraine is worse with activity in many patients so that diagnosis is in the differential, except in WD's case she does not meet the usual criteria for migraine with aura or migraine without aura. Also she was not on daily medications and thus medication overuse headache (MOH) as a cause of her headache can be excluded.

Secondary causes are present in about one third of exertional headache. On first occurrence of this headache type it is mandatory to exclude subarachnoid haemorrhage (SAH) and arterial dissection. In WD's case a CT scan and LP done after the presenting headache should serve as the basis for ruling out SAH, and if there were any question of dissection then a magnetic resonance angiogram (MRA) would be considered. The fact that her headache came on during a high velocity amusement ride would make it mandatory to undertake an MRI to rule out some of the rarer causes of secondary headache.

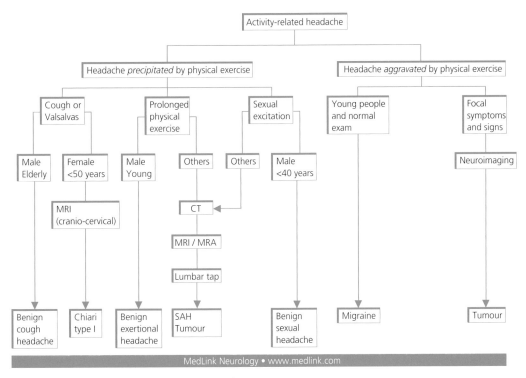

Figure 9.1 Flowhart of differential diagnosis of activity-related headache
Source: Pascual J. Activity-related headache. In *MedLink Neurology*. Ed S. Gilman San Diego: MedLink Corporation. Available at www.medlink.com. Accessed 10/12/2007.

Box 9.2 **International Classification of Headache Disorders. Diagnostic criteria for primary cough headache**

Previously used terms:
Benign cough headache, Valsalva-manoeuvre headache

Diagnostic criteria:
A. Headache fulfilling criteria B and C
B. Sudden onset, lasting from one second to 30 minutes
C. Brought on by and occurring only in association with coughing, straining and/or Valsalva manoeuvre
D. Not attributed to another disorder

Note: Cough headache is symptomatic in about 40% of cases and the large majority of these present Arnold-Chiari malformation type I. Other reported causes of symptomatic cough headache include carotid or vertebrobasilar diseases and cerebral aneurysms. Diagnostic neuroimaging plays an important role in differentiating secondary cough headache from primary cough headache.
Comment: Primary cough headache is usually bilateral and predominantly affects patients older than 40 years of age. Whilst indometacin is usually effective in the treatment of primary cough headache, a positive response to this medication has also been reported in some symptomatic cases.
Source: Headache Classification Subcommittee of the International Headache Society (IHS). *The International Classification of Headache Disorders* (2nd edition). *Cephalalgia* 2004; **24** (suppl 1): 1–160.

Box 9.3 **International Classification of Headache Disorders. Diagnostic criteria for primary headache associated with sexual activity**

Previously used terms:
Benign sex headache, coital cephalalgia, benign vascular sexual headache, sexual headache

Preorgasmic headache
Diagnostic criteria:
A. Dull ache in the head and neck associated with awareness of neck and/or jaw muscle contraction and meeting criterion B
B. Occurs during sexual activity and increases with sexual excitement
C. Not attributed to another disorder

Orgasmic headache
Diagnostic criteria:
A. Sudden severe ('explosive') headache meeting criterion B
B. Occurs at orgasm
C. Not attributed to another disorder

Note: On first onset of orgasmic headache it is mandatory to exclude condition such as subarachnoid haemorrhage and arterial dissection.
Comment: An association between primary headache associated with sexual activity, primary exertional headache and migraine is reported in approximately 50% of cases. No firm data are available on the duration of primary headache associated with sexual activity, but it is usually considered to last from 1 minute to 3 hours.
Source: adapted from Headache Classification Subcommittee of the International Headache Society (IHS). *The International Classification of Headache Disorders* (2nd edition). *Cephalalgia* 2004; **24**(suppl 1): 1–160.

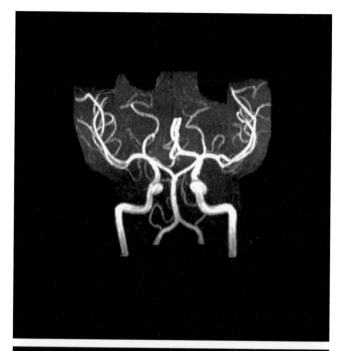

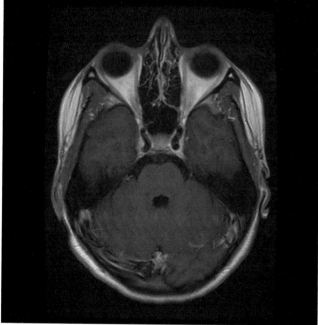

Figure 9.2 MRI scan showing MRA of normal cerebral and neck vessels, without aneurysm or dissection (2A) and MRI, with gadolinium enhancement showing no features of low pressure headache or intracranial carotid dissection (2B).

Preliminary diagnosis

The likely diagnosis in WD's case would be a secondary headache disorder as the features are not completely typical for primary exertional headache as symptoms are always present. SAH has been effectively ruled out and in this case there was a concern that a spinal fluid leak was producing her problem, since she said that the headache was worse when she stood up and better when she lay down prior to developing the headache. Thus an MRI scan was

Box 9.4 **International Classification of Headache Disorders. Diagnostic criteria for low cerebrospinal fluid pressure: CSF fistula headache**

Diagnostic criteria:

A. Headache that worsens within 15 minutes after sitting or standing, with at least one of the following and fulfilling criteria C and D:
   1. neck stiffness
   2. tinnitus
   3. hypacusia
   4. photophobia
   5. nausea
B. A known procedure or trauma has caused persistent CSF leakage with at least one of the following:
   1. evidence of low CSF pressure on MRI (e.g., pachymeningeal enhancement)
   2. evidence of CSF leakage on conventional myelography, CT myelography or cisternography
   3. CSF opening pressure <60 mm H_2O in sitting position
C. Headache develops in close temporal relation to CSF leakage
D. Headache resolves within 7 days of sealing the CSF leak

Source: adapted from Headache Classification Subcommittee of the International Headache Society (IHS). *The International Classification of Headache Disorders* (2nd edition). *Cephalalgia* 2004; **24** (suppl 1): 1–160.

done with gadolinium enhancement. It failed to demonstrate the classical features of low-pressure headache (Box 9.4) and an MRA was negative for dissection or intracranial aneurysm (Figure 9.2).

As no secondary cause had been found for her headaches, which were worse with exercise, then a diagnosis of primary exertional headache would have been appropriate.

Initial management

This includes:

- For primary exertional headache, moderation of activity is recommended and may be all that is necessary. If not, indometacin 50 mg three times a day has been found effective in the majority of the cases.
- WD should be advised to avoid frequent use, i.e. more than 15 days a month, of analgesics to prevent the evolution of medication overuse headache.

Other preventive treatment

Rarely other migraine preventive drugs medications have been used for primary exertional headache including: methysergide, propranolol, or flunarizine. Primary cough headaches usually respond to indometacin, and topiramate has shown some benefit in a few patients with cough headache.

Referral

If low-pressure headache were suspected (Box 9.4), referral to an anaesthetist with expertise in doing epidural blood patches would be appropriate. Referral is important in any case of CSF leak and if there is a secondary cause for the exertional headache or cough headache, such as a Chiari I malformation, then a neurosurgical opinion would be reasonable.

Final diagnosis

Primary exertional headache.

Outcome

WD was given indometacin to try to reduce or eliminate further exertional headaches. Importantly in this case the early recognition that there were atypical features to her story led to further investigation to rule out secondary causes of exertional headache. Although no secondary cause was found, such causes are worth looking for, as many are treatable. Long-term follow-up would be indicated in her case to ensure no secondary cause evolves, to ensure that she tolerates the treatments without serious side-effects, and that she avoids overuse of analgesic medication.

Further reading

Diamond S, Medina JL. Benign exertional headache: successful treatment with indomethacin. *Headache* 1979; **19**: 249.

Mathew NT. Indomethacin responsive headache syndromes. *Headache* 1981; **21**: 147–50.

Medrano V, Mallada J, Sempere AP, Fernández S, Piqueras L. Primary cough headache responsive to topiramate. *Cephalalgia* 2005; **25**: 627–8.

Mokri B. Spontaneous CSF leaks mimicking benign exertional headaches. *Cephalalgia* 2002; **22**: 780–3.

Pascual J, Iglesias F, Oterino A, Vázquez-Barquero A, Berciano J. Cough, exertional, and sexual headaches. An analysis of 72 benign and symptomatic cases. *Neurology* 1996; **46**: 1520–4.

Rooke ED. Benign exertional headache. *Med Clin North Am* 1968; **52**: 801–8.

Sjaastad O, Bakketeig LS. Exertional headache. I. Vaga study of headache epidemiology. *Cephalalgia* 2002; **22**: 784–90.

Sjaastad O, Bakketeig LS. Prolonged benign exertional headache. The Vaga study of headache epidemiology. *Headache* 2003; **43**: 611–15.

CHAPTER 10

Thunderclap Headache

David W. Dodick

OVERVIEW

- All patients presenting with a worrisome headache must be questioned about the acuity of onset and time-to-peak intensity of the headache
- Thunderclap headache may be idiopathic or symptomatic of sinister intracranial pathology
- All patients with thunderclap headache must be thoroughly investigated, including cerebrovascular imaging, for all conditions which can cause sudden severe headache

CASE HISTORY

The man with a sudden severe headache
JR is a 42-year-old male presenting to the Emergency Department with a severe headache associated with nausea, photophobia and recurrent vomiting. The headache is occipital, began while straining at stool, and has persisted for the last three hours. He prefers to lie still as activity or minimal exertion worsens the headache. He has a 12-year history of episodic migraine and usually experiences about two attacks a year. This headache is more severe and began more suddenly than his previous migraine headaches.

History

How many different headache types does the patient experience?

JR has two headache types. He has a 12-year history of episodic migraine without aura and the headache with which he now presents, which he believes is different from any migraine attack he has ever had. His migraine attacks are usually unilateral, intensify gradually over 1–2 hours, and are moderate in severity. This headache is much more severe, began suddenly while straining at stool, and is mainly occipital in location. He has also vomited twice with this headache, and while he sometimes experiences nausea with his migraine attacks, he has never vomited.

Time questions

The pain is extremely severe and the onset of the headache was very sudden. The pain peaked almost instantaneously while strain-

ing at stool. The time to peak intensity was less than 20 seconds. The headache has persisted without relief for the past three hours.

Character questions

The headache began and remains confined to the occipital region. It is associated with photophobia, nausea and emesis. He feels flushed but is not febrile. There is no neck stiffness, changes in vision or focal neurological symptoms. The pain was not preceded by premonitory or aura symptoms. The pain is worsened with straining and routine physical activity.

Cause questions

The precipitating factor in this case appeared to be straining at stool. This is the first time JR has experienced this type of headache. Previous migraine attacks were not triggered by a Valsalva manoeuvre. There is no family history of similar headaches, though there is a family history of migraine without aura in JR's mother, maternal aunts and maternal grandmother.

Response to headache questions

The patient has not been able to function since the onset of this headache because of its severity. He has tried ibuprofen 600 mg and acetaminophen 1300 mg without relief. This may be partly due to lack of absorption due to recurrent emesis.

State of health between attacks

JR has been in good health prior to the onset of this headache. Other than migraine without aura, he has no significant past medical history, does not regularly take medications or supplements, and does not use illicit drugs. He drinks 1–2 glasses of wine with dinner each evening, but does not drink alcohol to excess.

Examination

JR is alert and his mental state is normal. Blood pressure is 162/96 mmHg, heart rate 90 beats per minute, respirations 20 per minute, and temperature is 36.2° Celsius. He is lying on his side, both hands on his head, and is in obvious discomfort. Neurological examination is normal. Fundi were well visualized and without abnormality. Neck was supple, without meningismus.

ABC of Headache. Edited by A. MacGregor & A. Frith.
© 2009 Blackwell Publishing, ISBN 978-1-4051-7066-6.

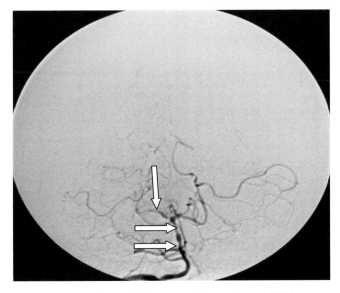

Figure 10.1 Reversible cerebral vasoconstriction syndrome. Multiple areas of segmental vasoconstriction in the posterior circulation are evident

Box 10.1 **Differential diagnosis of thunderclap headache**

Vascular
- Subarachnoid haemorrhage
- Cerebral venous sinus thrombosis*
- Cervical artery (carotid or vertebral) dissection*
- Reversible cerebral vasoconstriction syndrome*
- Acute hypertensive crisis*
- Ischaemic stroke
- Pituitary apoplexy*

Non-vascular
- Spontaneous CSF leak*
- Colloid cyst of the third ventricle

Primary headache disorders
- Primary cough headache
- Primary exertional headache
- Primary sexual headache
- Primary thunderclap headache

*Disorders sometimes or often undetected on routine non-contrast head CT.

Investigations

JR's complete blood count, serum chemistry, urinalysis, urine drug screen and electrocardiogram revealed no abnormalities or remarkable findings. Unenhanced brain CT was normal. There was no evidence of subarachnoid haemorrhage, ischaemic or intraparenchymal haemorrhagic stroke or intracranial mass lesion. Lumbar puncture revealed opening pressure 12 cm water, CSF was clear and without red or white blood cells, xanthochromia, and serum-matched total protein and glucose were normal. Gram stain was negative. Brain MRI, MR venography and MR angiography revealed multiple areas of vasoconstriction involving the anterior and posterior cerebral arteries (Figure 10.1).

Diagnosis

Differential diagnosis

The differential diagnosis of thunderclap headache (TCH) is one of the most important in medicine because of the morbidity and mortality associated with the conditions that can present with TCH. Immediate referral to the Emergency Department is warranted. The diagnosis may be challenging, especially when the headache occurs in isolation and in the absence of neurological symptoms or signs, thereby lowering the index of suspicion of a sinister secondary cause. The diagnosis is made even more challenging because many of the secondary causes may not be detected on the initial investigations such as computed tomography of the brain and lumbar puncture.

The differential diagnosis consists of both primary and secondary headache disorders (Box 10.1). The clinical approach to the patient with thunderclap headache should be methodical and should be tailored to evaluate each of these causes in an appropriate and sequential fashion (Figure 10.2). It is evident from the differential diagnosis that a number of secondary causes may not be detected on routine brain CT or lumbar puncture and therefore additional imaging studies are required when these initial investigations are unrevealing.

Preliminary diagnosis

Reversible cerebral vasoconstriction syndrome (RCVS). RCVS consists of a group of disorders characterized by reversible segmental cerebral vasoconstriction (Box 10.2).

In the absence of a defined precipitating disease or drug, the syndrome is triggered by a Valsalva manoeuvre in approximately 90% of patients. It is likely a commonly overlooked cause for thunderclap headache, as recent studies indicate that 40–60% of patients who present with TCH and a negative CT and LP have cerebral vasoconstriction when MR angiography is performed. Patients usually present with isolated TCH, but may present or develop associated symptoms such as altered cognition, motor and sensory deficits, seizures, visual disturbances, ataxia, speech abnormalities, nausea and vomiting. RCVS must be considered in patients who present with TCH, vasoconstriction of one or more arteries of the cerebral arteries that constitute the circle of Willis, and normal or near-normal cerebrospinal fluid. The lack of cortical and subcortical infarctions at presentation and the normal spinal fluid distinguish this syndrome from CNS vasculitis. Rapid and accurate diagnosis is important, however, since ischaemic or haemorrhage stroke may occur in up to one third of patients in the following weeks and treatment with calcium channel blockers may be effective in reversing the vasoconstriction and minimizing the risk of stroke.

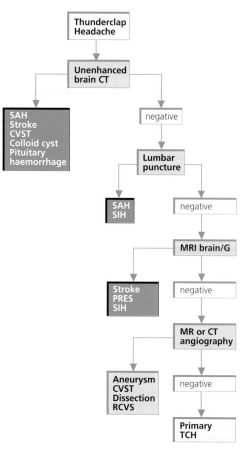

Figure 10.2 Clinical algorithm for the evaluation of thunderclap headache CVST: cerebral venous sinus thrombosis; MRI brain/G: with gadolinium; PRES: posterior reversible encephalopathy syndrome usually due to hypertensive crisis; RCVS: reversible cerebral vasoconstriction syndrome; SAH: subarachnoid haemorrhage; SIH: spontaneous intracranial hypotension secondary to CSF leak; TCH: thunderclap headache. Source: adapted with permission from Schwedt TJ, Matharu MS, Dodick DW. Thunderclap headache. *Lancet Neurol* 2006; **5(7)**: 621–31.

Initial management

This includes judicious management of blood pressure, hydration, headache treatment with analgesics, avoidance of drugs with vaso-constrictor activity (e.g. triptans, ergots) and initiation of calcium channel blockers. Rapid decrease in blood pressure is generally not recommended in the presence of vasoconstriction because of the risk of compromising cerebral blood flow beyond a severe constric-tion in a major cerebral artery. Nimodipine and verapamil have been reported to be effective, though there have been no controlled clinical trials. Treatment is therefore empiric and cannot be guided by a robust literature or consensus.

Nimodipine is usually initiated at a dose of 30–60 mg every six hours for a period of two weeks at which point vascular imaging, either with CT angiography or MR angiography, is repeated to demonstrate reversal of vasoconstriction. Reversal of angiographic

---

> **Box 10.2 Conditions associated with reversible cerebral vasoconstriction syndrome**
>
> - Pregnancy, eclampsia, pre-eclampsia, early puerperium
> - Exposure to drugs and blood products (e.g. bromocriptine, SSRIs, sumatriptan, cocaine, intravenous immunoglobulin, pseudoephedrine, phenylpropanolamine, ecstasy, triptans, methergine, ergotamine)
> - Miscellaneous (e.g. pheochromocytoma, carotid endarterectomy, hypercalcemia, porphyria, bronchial carcinoid tumour)
> - Valsalva manoeuvre (cough, physical exertion, strain, sexual activity, etc.)

findings is usually present at 2–4 weeks after the onset of headache, but may take up to two months to reverse fully. Nimodipine is continued until reversibility has been demonstrated and the patient is asymptomatic, without headache or any associated symptoms, for at least seven days.

Referral

Referral should be considered in the patient where CNS vasculitis is suspected, neurological symptoms develop or evidence of rever-sal of vasoconstriction is not evident within a two-month period.

Final diagnosis

Reversible cerebral vasoconstriction syndrome.

Management plan

Long-term treatment is not required. Recurrence appears to be rare.

Outcome

JR experienced recurrent thunderclap headaches over the next two days. Blood pressure was not managed with medications and nor-malized without treatment. Nimodipine was initiated at a dose of 60 mg every six hours for the first week, then 30 mg every six hours for the next three weeks. MR angiogram of the head and neck was repeated four weeks after the first imaging study and demonstrated complete resolution of the cerebral vasoconstriction.

Further reading

Calabrese LH, Dodick DW, Schwedt TJ, Singhal AB. Reversible cerebral vaso-constriction syndromes. *Ann Int Med* 2007; **146(1)**: 34–44.

Chen SP, Fuh JL, Lirng JF, Chang FC, Wang SJ. Recurrent primary thunder-clap headache and benign CNS angiopathy: spectra of the same disorder? *Neurology* 2006; **67(12)**: 2164–9.

Schwedt TJ, Matharu MS, Dodick DW. Thunderclap headache. *Lancet Neurol* 2006; **5(7)**: 621–31.

CHAPTER 11

Headache and Brain Tumour

R. Allan Purdy

OVERVIEW

- History is important to confirm the headache is not secondary to another causation
- Secondary headaches can present as mimics of primary headaches
- Patients with seizures can have headaches
- Management must take into account headaches and causation of symptoms

CASE HISTORY

The woman with headaches and hallucinations

KM is a 46-year-old woman with a lifelong history of headache that is worse with menses. Her headaches are unilateral in the temple, worse with movement, better with rest, lasting part of a day and worse with bright lights, sounds and sometimes smell. She rarely has an aura and, when present, it is visual with zigzag lines on one side of her vision.

She presented one day at the Emergency Department with severe headache in the right parietal area and felt a jolt in that area with movement. She had visual and auditory hallucinations persisting for 24 hours. She was admitted in status migrainosus and treated. Neurological examination was completely normal.

History

How many different headache types does the patient experience?

KM has three types of headache. She has a long history of migraine without aura and sometimes with aura. She also had a new severe parietal headache associated with unusual symptoms and hallucinations of undetermined cause, although this was thought to be status migrainosus.

Time questions

KM has a life-long history of recurrent, severe headache, worse with menses and sometimes with classic visual aura which is forti-

fication spectra or zigzag lines. This suggests a benign aetiology and primary headache disorder. The change to a more severe and atypical headache clinically, despite a normal examination, is worrisome, as is any changing headache.

Character questions

Migraine is usually a moderate to severe headache. Her new headache was also severe – something that could occur in status migrainosus or migraine occurring daily and unabated. Thus severity alone is not the clinical characteristic that raises suspicion.

Cause questions

It is important to determine the mechanism of the head jolt as this symptom is rare in migraine. However, sharp jabs and jolts can occur in other primary headache disorders, including primary stabbing headache and the paroxysmal hemicranias. Other symptoms atypical for migraine are the hallucinatory phenomena and the duration of the neurological symptoms, which should not last 24 hours.

Response to headache questions

KM admitted that the last headache was different from her usual migraine headache. The visual symptoms were also different, in that she saw increased trails on images moving across the visual field. In addition, she was hearing voices.

State of health between attacks

KM was well between her headaches over the years, but with the recent change in headache she began to have more aura in terms of the recurrent visual and auditory hallucinations.

Examination

Her neurological examination was normal, as were her vital signs and general examination.

Investigations

KM had a CT scan, which showed some attenuation in the white matter of her right temporal lobe but no mass effect or other intracranial changes. An MRI scan and EEG were arranged. Her routine blood tests in the Emergency Department were normal.

ABC of Headache. Edited by A. MacGregor & A. Frith.
© 2009 Blackwell Publishing, ISBN 978-1-4051-7066-6.

Diagnosis

Differential diagnosis

This history is worrisome because of the change of headache characteristics, new symptoms of hallucinosis and head jolt, and the fact the headache was different from prior migraine. Thus this case has the major 'red flags' (Box 11.1) of the changing headache: her neurological symptoms became prolonged and hallucinosis would be unusual in migraine, especially occurring many years after onset.

These symptoms, despite the normal examination, are of concern; however, with the addition of a focal white matter change in the right temporal lobe, the diagnosis must exclude a secondary cause of headache, including a neoplasm. White matter lesions are increasingly being seen on neuroimaging of migraine patients, particularly MRI scans. This case requires careful follow-up and repeat imaging.

Preliminary diagnosis

KM continued to be asymptomatic between attacks, but an unenhanced MRI scan showed a white matter lesion in the right temporal lobe (Figure 11.1). This was believed to represent a migraine white matter lesion or an early neoplasm of probably white matter in nature. Importantly, no other white matter lesions were seen. So the working diagnosis was a) migraine with and without aura, and b) headache and white matter lesion not yet diagnosed, possibly migraine or other, possible tumour?

It should be noted that the headache of brain tumour is non-specific and may resemble tension-type headache, migraine headache or other headache types. Important facts about headache and brain tumour are outlined in Box 11.2.

Initial management

Initial management is shown in Box 11.3.

Explanation to patient

In headache medicine it is vital that patients fully understand the nature of their headaches, the causes if known, the treatments proposed and the need for follow-up. In KM's case it was relatively easy to diagnose and manage her migraine headaches. What was difficult was the diagnostic uncertainty around the other headache

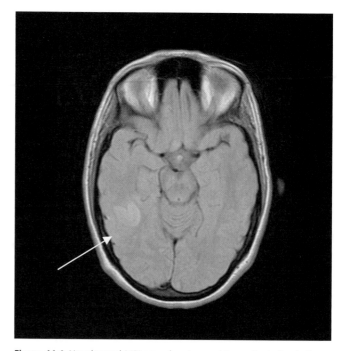

Figure 11.1 Unenhanced MRI scan showing a white matter lesion in the right temporal lobe

and neurological symptoms in light of the MR finding. Nevertheless, a frank discussion at this point, including the possibility that there might be a neoplasm, was accepted, as was the need for careful follow-up.

Treatment with migraine-specific medications

Treatment of her acute migraine attacks involved avoidance of triggers, including bright lights and loud sounds, however moder-

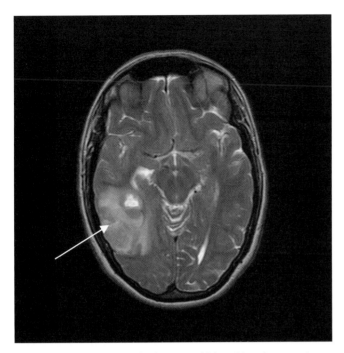

Figure 11.2 Enhanced MRI of right temporal lobe with oedema consistent with a neoplasm

ate to severe headache would probably require intervention with medication. In KM's case she responded well to a triptan taken early in the attack. She also took naproxen sodium for her menstrual migraine and a triptan as well. She was told she could use an anti-emetic such as metoclopramide for nausea and vomiting and if her 'migraine' became severe again then further parenteral therapy might be used, including prochlorperazine/metoclopramide and steroids. Fortunately, KM did not need these therapies as her migraine responded well to a triptan.

EEG

KM had an outpatient EEG. This showed slowing over the right temporal lobe in the form of a focal delta rhythm, but no epileptiform activity. This was a worrisome finding because of the lateralization of the slowing and the fact that focal slowing is frequently indicative of a structural lesion. An EEG was ordered because of the hallucinations and to determine if these were the result of recurrent partial simple seizures rather than migraine. The fact there was slowing, even in the absence of seizure activity, was ominous and suggested the hallucinations were in fact seizures.

It should be noted that in most headache patients EEG is not necessary, and in migraine dysrhythmia may be seen. There are also cases of migralepsy where migraine and seizures occur together, but without focal lesions.

Repeat MRI head scan with gadolinium enhancement

This was the key test in KM's case. When repeated shortly after the EEG and three months after her presentation in the Emergency

Department, it showed a significant white matter lesion in her right temporal lobe with oedema, consistent with a neoplasm (Figure 11.2).

Follow-up

KM was to return to the clinic for follow-up. However, prior to that appointment her hallucinosis increased, along with her right-sided headache, and she developed nausea and vomiting. She was seen urgently, and a repeat CT scan with enhancement showed a large mass lesion in the right temporal lobe with oedema consistent with a malignant brain tumour. Her examination at this time remained normal, although she was drowsy and in distress because of her headache and neurological symptoms.

Referral

KM was referred to neurosurgery, where a right temporal lobe biopsy was arranged and revealed a malignant glioblastoma multiforme.

Final diagnosis

Migraine with and without aura, and glioblastoma multiforme with headache and partial simple seizures.

Management plan

KM was started on dexamethasone 4 mg four times daily. This gave good relief of her headache and she was more alert. She was also loaded with intravenous diphenylhydantoin and subsequently had a marked reduction in her hallucinosis.

Outcome

KM remained symptom-free, except for an occasional migraine headache, without other major symptoms for the next couple of months. She received radiation therapy for her tumour. After two months she became drowsy and obtunded and was hospitalized with return of the non-migraine headache. Conservative therapy was requested by the family based on the patient's prior wishes. She slipped into coma and died three days later.

Further reading

Forsyth PA, Posner JB. Headaches in patients with brain tumors: a study of 111 patients. *Neurology* 1992; **43**: 1678–83.

Kruit MC, van Buchem MA, Hofman PAM, et al. Migraine as a risk factor for subclinical brain lesions. *JAMA* 2004; **291**(4): 427–34.

Purdy RA, Kirby S. Headache and brain tumors. *Neurol Clin N Am* 2004; **22**: 39–53.

Silberstein SD, Lipton RB, Dalessio DJ. *Wolff's Headache's and Other Head Pains*. Oxford: Oxford University Press, 2001.

CHAPTER 12

Headache and Neck Pain

Anne MacGregor

CASE HISTORY

The man with a painful neck
AS is a 43-year-old banker. He presents with recurrent neck and head pain, aggravated by movement of the neck. Initially episodic, he now has pain most of the time. The pain does not prevent his daily activities, but it is beginning to interfere with his work.

History

How many different headache types does the patient experience?

AS responds that he gets the occasional hangover, but otherwise his only headache is from his neck.

Time questions

The headache started a couple of years ago but only occurred after AS had been working at his computer for extended periods of time. It has become more frequent over the last year and lasts most of the day. It tends to build up over the week and eases during the weekend.

Character questions

The intensity can vary from mild to moderate. It is a constant, non-throbbing pain with no associated symptoms and no upper limb symptoms. AS points to where the pain starts, in the right side of the neck. He moves his hand up the neck over the head as he describes how the pain spreads up into the right occipital and parietal regions as well as into the right shoulder.

ABC of Headache. Edited by A. MacGregor & A. Frith.
© 2009 Blackwell Publishing, ISBN 978-1-4051-7066-6.

Cause questions

AS used to find that massage helped, but then it started to aggravate the pain. He finds that getting up from his desk and moving can lessen the symptoms. He used to swim at weekends, which helped. He has stopped swimming over recent months, as he no longer has the time. The pain is much worse if he does not take regular breaks from the computer. He had a whiplash injury five years ago and thinks that this may be the cause.

Response to headache questions

AS tried paracetamol, which would ease the pain for a while, but he stopped taking it as he did not want to rely on painkillers. He tried a triptan, given to him by a locum doctor who had diagnosed migraine, but it did not have any effect. He saw a sports physiotherapist who gave him some exercises to try. Although these helped, he did not have time to continue treatment.

State of health between attacks

Aside from the headaches, AS has no other medical problems.

Examination

AS is normotensive. Physical and brief neurological examination is unremarkable, except for limited lateral flexion of the neck, particularly to the right. Longus colli and trapezius muscles are increased in tone and tender to palpation, particularly on the right. There are no neurological signs.

Investigations

The history and examination do not suggest a need for further investigation. Given his age, AS is likely to have degenerative changes on plain radiographs of the cervical spine, which correlate poorly with clinical symptoms and are just as likely to be found in asymptomatic people (Figure 12.1). If rheumatoid arthritis is suspected, flexion and extension radiographs of the neck will identify severe atlanto-axial subluxation. If more serious pathology is suspected, magnetic resonance imaging of the cervical spine is the investigation of choice, as it gives detailed information. If there is evidence of systemic illness, additional investigations such as full blood count, erythrocyte sedimentation rate, C-reactive protein

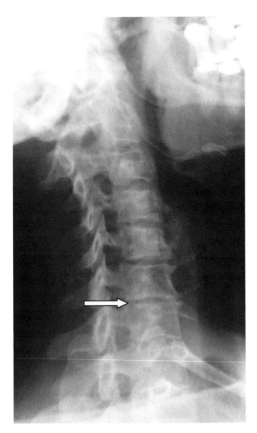

Figure 12.1 Oblique radiograph of the cervical spine in a patient with cervical spondylosis showing loss of disc height, anterior osteophytosis and narrowing of the foramina
Source: Binder AI. Clinical review: Cervical spondylosis and neck pain. *BMJ* 2007; **334**: 527–31.

Table 12.1 Cervical diseases causing headache*

Congenital	Developmental anomalies, e.g. congenital atlantoaxial dislocation
Traumatic	Rotatory subluxation of the atlas
Inflammatory	Osteomyelitis
Neoplastic	Multiple myeloma
	Tumours, e.g. meningioma, schwannoma, ependymoma
Endocrine/metabolic	Paget's disease
Autoimmune	Rheumatoid arthritis
Psychological	Psychogenic headache

*Whiplash and degenerative changes are not accepted as causes of chronic headache.

and protein electrophoresis should be considered to exclude other pathologies.

Diagnosis

Differential diagnosis

Several cervical structures are pain-sensitive (Box 12.1). Any condition that affects these structures can give rise to headache (Table 12.1). AS has no 'red flag' features to suggest underlying disease (Box 12.2). Nor does he experience suggestive features of craniovertebral abnormalities such as Arnold-Chiari malformation, which would include posterior location, triggered by neck flexion or coughing and straining, or a pronounced postural effect. In the absence of these, the main differential diagnosis is tension-type headache and migraine, both of which may present with coexisting neck pain, and cervicogenic headache (Figure 12.2).

Migraine is unlikely given the duration of attacks and absence of associated symptoms. Tension-type headache is possible, although the pain is typically bilateral, mild to moderate and described as pressing or squeezing. Nausea, photophobia, phonophobia, dizziness, blurred vision and dysphagia are occasionally present with tension-type headache, but the symptoms are not pronounced.

Box 12.2 **'Red flag' features and the conditions they suggest**

Malignancy, infection or inflammation
- Fever, night sweats
- Unexplained weight loss
- History of inflammatory arthritis, malignancy, infection, tuberculosis, HIV infection, drug dependency or immunosuppression
- Excruciating pain
- Intractable night pain
- Cervical lymphadenopathy
- Exquisite tenderness over a vertebral body

Myelopathy
- Gait disturbance or clumsy hands, or both
- Objective neurological deficit – upper motor neurone signs in the legs and lower motor neurone signs in the arms
- Sudden onset in a young patient suggests disc prolapse

Other
- History of severe osteoporosis
- History of neck surgery
- Drop attacks, especially when moving the neck, suggest vascular disease
- Intractable or increasing pain

Source: Binder AI. Clinical review: cervical spondylosis and neck pain. *BMJ* 2007; **334**: 527–31.

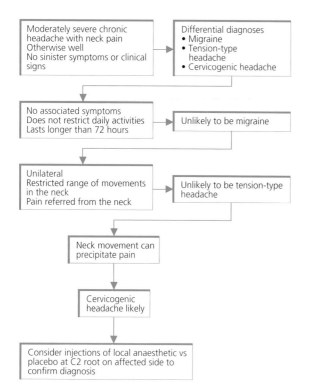

Figure 12.2 Flowchart of differential diagnosis

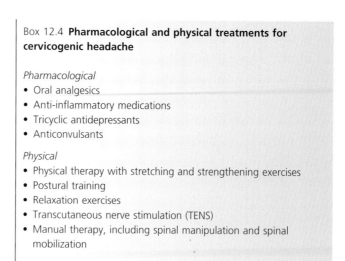

Box 12.4 **Pharmacological and physical treatments for cervicogenic headache**

Pharmacological
- Oral analgesics
- Anti-inflammatory medications
- Tricyclic antidepressants
- Anticonvulsants

Physical
- Physical therapy with stretching and strengthening exercises
- Postural training
- Relaxation exercises
- Transcutaneous nerve stimulation (TENS)
- Manual therapy, including spinal manipulation and spinal mobilization

Further evidence is that external pressure over the upper cervical or occipital region on the affected side precipitates pain. The headache is characterized by continuous, unilateral head pain radiating from the occipital areas to the frontal area, with associated neck pain and ipsilateral shoulder or arm pain. It is described as a dull, non-throbbing, boring, dragging pain that can fluctuate in intensity. The headache can last from a few hours to several days and, in some cases, several weeks. A recent or past history of head or neck trauma is common but does not contribute to the diagnosis. Cervicogenic headache affects four times as many women as men, the majority being in their early 40s.

Initial management

This includes reassurance and symptomatic treatment.

Numerous treatments for cervicogenic headache have been attempted, with varying levels of success (Box 12.4). Pharmacological treatments such as muscle relaxants can give short-term relief, but are associated with side-effects and are not recommended for long-term use. AS does not want to take medication as he is concerned that it might impair his work. Given the structural basis of the pain, physical treatments are more successful in treating the underlying cause.

Referral

There is no indication for routine referral. In accordance with the International Headache Society, the diagnosis could be confirmed by injections of local anaesthetic and placebo at the C2 root on the affected side. These injections should be given one week apart. Abolition of headache should follow injection with the local anaesthetic but not with placebo. Since AS's headache can be precipitated by movement of the neck, this approach is unnecessary but could be considered if the diagnosis was uncertain.

Final diagnosis

Cervicogenic headache.

Box 12.3 **International Classification of Headache Disorders. Diagnostic criteria for cervicogenic headache**

Diagnostic criteria
A. Pain, referred from a source in the neck and perceived in one or more regions of the head and/or face, fulfilling criteria C and D
B. Clinical, laboratory and/or imaging evidence of a disorder or lesion within the cervical spine or soft tissues of the neck known to be, or generally accepted as, a valid cause of headache
C. Evidence that the pain can be attributed to the neck disorder or lesion based on at least one of the following:
   1. demonstration of clinical signs that implicate a source of pain in the neck
   2. abolition of headache following diagnostic blockade of a cervical structure or its nerve supply using placebo or other adequate controls
D. Pain resolves within three months of successful treatment of the causative disorder or lesion

Source: Headache Classification Subcommittee of the International Headache Society (IHS). *The International Classification of Headache Disorders* (2nd edition). *Cephalalgia* 2004; **24** (suppl 1): 1–160.

Preliminary diagnosis

Cervicogenic headache should be considered if neck movement precipitates headache, particularly if there is also restricted range of motion in the neck (Box 12.3).

Management plan

AS is given advice on stress management and time planning. He is offered spinal manipulation but chooses to return to the sports physiotherapist with the aim to improve muscular strength in the neck and shoulders. AS recognizes that his lifestyle has contributed significantly to the problem and plans to start a regular exercise programme. His workstation is reviewed to reduce ergonomic problems. He gets a headset to replace the hand-held phone, which he uses frequently throughout the day. He repositions his monitor so that it is placed directly in front of him to avoid excessive twisting of the neck. He adjusts the height of his chair until his feet can rest flat on the floor.

Outcome

Having identified the physical nature of this headache, simple strategies to alleviate the cause and prevent the problem recurring are successful. AS's headache gradually improved over a couple of months. It occasionally recurs if he works for extended periods at his computer, but since he understands the cause of the headache, he is able to treat it by making sure he takes regular breaks.

Further reading

Binder AI. Clinical review: cervical spondylosis and neck pain. *BMJ* 2007; **334**: 527–31.

Bogduk N. The neck and headaches. *Neurol Clin* 2004; **22**(1): 151–71.

Edmeads J. The cervical spine and headache. *Neurology* 1988; **38**: 1874–8.

Göbel H, Edmeads JG. Disorders of the skull and cervical spine. In: Olesen J, Goadsby PJ, Ramadan N, Tfelt-Hansen P, Welch KMA (Eds). *The Headaches*. 3rd edition. Philadelphia: Lippincott Williams & Wilkins, **2006**: 1003–11.

CHAPTER 13

Headache and Depression

Anne MacGregor

OVERVIEW

- Primary headaches and depression are co-morbid conditions
- Frequent headaches should prompt evaluation of depression
- Most depression can be managed in primary care
- Patients with treatment-resistant, recurrent, atypical and psychotic depression, or who have significant suicide risk, should be referred to a mental health specialist

CASE HISTORY

The woman with daily headache
SF is a 40-year-old teacher who has had 'sick' headaches associated with menstruation since the age of 23. These were diagnosed as menstrual migraine and she has usually been able to control them with symptomatic treatments. She is seeking help because the attacks have become much longer, more frequent and less responsive to treatment.

History

How many different headache types does the patient experience?

On direct questioning, SF reports that she has typical menstrual migraines. She has also had a different type of headache a couple of times a week. This pattern of headaches is confirmed by three months of diaries.

Time questions

Although SF used to get occasional headaches outside of her periods, she is now getting them two or three times a week and they last most of the day. Menstrual migraines now last between five and seven days a month.

Character questions

Menstrual migraines are moderate to severe throbbing headaches associated with nausea, vomiting, photophobia and phonophobia. The second type of headache SF describes as more like pressure, or

ABC of Headache. Edited by A. MacGregor & A. Frith.
© 2009 Blackwell Publishing, ISBN 978-1-4051-7066-6.

a heavy weight on her head as if she were wearing a heavy helmet. There are no associated symptoms.

Cause questions

Although the menstrual migraines have an obvious cause, SF is unable to identify any reason why they were more severe. Her periods have not changed in any way. She mentions that there have been some problems at work recently and wonders if this could be causing the other headaches.

Response to headache questions

SF is now losing a couple of days a month because of menstrual migraines. She takes sumatriptan 50 mg at the start of the attack, but this is not as effective as in the past and she is confined to bed. Symptoms typically recur on several consecutive days and it is not until the third day that sumatriptan takes effect and she can return to work. She tried treating the pressure headaches with painkillers but they did not make any difference so she stopped using them. The headaches do not prevent her going to work, but she finds it difficult to concentrate and worries about making mistakes.

State of health between attacks

When asked about how she feels when she does not have a headache, SF becomes tearful. She mentions that she had similar headaches a couple of years ago, which she put down to her job at the time, which she hated. She resigned and started a new job a year ago, which had been going well until a new, more senior colleague started six months ago. This colleague is very critical and unsupportive and SF is finding it increasingly difficult to cope. This has become worse now that SF is losing one or two days a month through migraine.

SF feels controlled by her headaches. She is finding it difficult to sleep, waking early in the morning and feeling tired all the time. This is much worse just before her period, when she feels bloated and irritable. When asked if she is depressed, she becomes angry, denying any past or current history of depression. She says that when she was a child, she remembers her mother, who also had migraine, being treated for depression. She states, 'I'm not like my mother and if someone just sorted my periods out, I'd be fine.'

In response to the question 'During the last month, have you often been bothered by having little interest or pleasure in doing things?' SF replies, 'Most of the time.' On further questioning, she reveals that she split up with her partner two months ago, when she found out that he was having an affair. She is upset about not having children and feels that time is running out. She feels that no one wants to be with her and she avoids social occasions.

Remaining medical history is unremarkable. There are no symptoms of any underlying medical disorder. SF denies alcohol or substance abuse and has no suicidal thoughts. She is not taking any medication other than sumatriptan and a liquid iron supplement, which she has taken for several years.

Examination

BP 125/80 and her pulse is a regular 72 beats per minute. Funduscopy and brief physical and neurological examination are unremarkable.

Investigations

As there are no sinister symptoms in the history and no abnormal findings on physical examination, there is no indication for further investigation at this stage.

Diagnosis

Differential diagnosis

SF has herself identified two different headaches: menstrual migraine (see chapter 6) and a second, more frequent headache suggestive of episodic tension-type headache (see chapter 3). Patients with depression often present with somatic complaints that mask the underlying depression. Despite her denial, SF presents with three key symptoms of depression and two associated symptoms (disturbed sleep, low self-confidence) suggesting moderate depression (Box 13.1).

Physical and somatic symptoms can be quickly assessed using the Patient Health Questionnaire (PHQ-9). This self-administered questionnaire consists of nine items correlating to the DSM-IV diagnostic criteria and is a validated method of detecting and quantifying the severity of depression (Box 13.2). It can also be used to monitor the response to treatment.

Numerous studies have shown co-morbidity between depression and primary headache. It is not clear if depression is a consequence of frequent headache, or if headache is a symptom of depression. Evidence suggests dysregulation in serotonergic and noradrenergic pathways, and in nociception, may underlie both conditions, confirming their organic basis.

Whatever the association, depression needs to be fully evaluated. The first step in management is to exclude underlying medical conditions as a cause. These include inter-current viral infection, endocrine disorders such as hypothroidism, and neoplasia. If a physical cause for the depression is ruled out, a psychological evaluation should be done. This should include a complete history of symptoms – when they started, how long they have lasted, how severe they are, whether the patient had them before and, if so, whether the symptoms were treated and what treatment was given.

It is important to assess risk of suicide (Box 13.3). Family history of depression should be elicited and, if treated, what treatments were used and which were effective.

SF has no significant clinical symptoms or signs to suggest an underlying medical disorder. There is no evidence of medication overuse on the history or on review of the diary cards.

Box 13.1 **Assessing depression**

Key symptoms
   persistent sadness or low mood; and/or
   loss of interests or pleasure
   fatigue or low energy
At least one of these, most days, most of the time for at least two weeks.

If any of above present, ask about associated symptoms
   disturbed sleep
   poor concentration or indecisiveness
   low self-confidence
   poor or increased appetite
   suicidal thoughts or acts
   agitation or slowing of movements
   guilt or self-blame

Then ask about past, family history, associated disability and availability of social support
1. Factors that favour general advice and watchful waiting
      four or fewer of the above symptoms
      no past or family history
      social support available
      symptoms intermittent, or less than two weeks
      not actively suicidal
      little associated disability
2. Factors that favour more active treatment in primary care
      five or more symptoms
      past history or family history of depression
      low social support
      suicidal thoughts
      associated social disability
3. Factors that favour referral to mental health professionals
      poor or incomplete response to two interventions
      recurrent episode within one year of last one
      patient or relatives request referral
      self-neglect
4. Factors that favour urgent referral to a psychiatrist
      actively suicidal ideas or plans
      psychotic symptoms
      severe agitation accompanying severe (more than 10) symptoms
      severe self-neglect

ICD-10 definitions
Mild depression: four symptoms
Moderate depression: five or six symptoms
Severe depression: seven or more symptoms, with or without psychotic features

Preliminary diagnosis
1. Menstrually-related migraine without aura
2. Episodic tension-type headache
3. Moderate depression

Box 13.2 **Patient Health Questionnaire (PHQ-9)**

Patient Name _____ **Date** _____

1. **Over the last 2 weeks, how often have you been bothered by any of the following problems? Read each item carefully, and tick your response.**

	Not at all	Several days	More than half the days	Nearly every day
	0	1	2	3
a. Little interest or pleasure in doing things				
b. Feeling down, depressed, or hopeless				
c. Trouble falling asleep, staying asleep, or sleeping too much				
d. Feeling tired or having little energy				
e. Poor appetite or overeating				
f. Feeling bad about yourself, feeling that you are a failure, or feeling that you have let yourself or your family down				
g. Trouble concentrating on things such as reading the newspaper or watching television				
h. Moving or speaking so slowly that other people could have noticed. Or being so fidgety or restless that you have been moving around a lot more than usual				
i. Thinking that you would be better off dead or that you want to hurt yourself in some way				
Totals				

2. **If you checked off any problem on this questionnaire so far, how difficult have these problems made it for you to do your work, take care of things at home, or get along with other people?**

Not Difficult At All	Somewhat Difficult	Very Difficult	Extremely Difficult
0	1	2	3

SCORE:

Question 1

0–4	No or minimal depression
5–9	Mild depression
10–14	Moderate depression
15–19	Moderately severe depression
≥20	Severe depression

Question Two

The responses 'very difficult' or 'extremely difficult' suggest that the patient's functionality is impaired.

Initial management

When several disorders coexist, review each separately. For SF, acute treatment of the menstrual migraine is inadequate. One option is to increase sumatriptan to 100 mg, taken in combination with naproxen 250–500 mg. Another is to consider management strategies that would benefit both coexisting disorders, using a treatment for depression that is also a prophylactic for migraine and headache.

SF resists the suggestion that she is depressed as she considers depression a sign of a weakness. With careful explanation of the biological nature of depression, she begins to accept the diagnosis. For moderate depression, antidepressant medication is offered (Figure 13.1). Selective serotonin reuptake inhibitors (SSRIs) are as effective as tricyclic antidepressants and less likely to be discontinued because of anticholinergic and sedative side-effects (Table 13.1). However, the only antidepressant with established efficacy in the prevention of primary headache is the tricyclic drug amitriptyline (Table 13.2). SF asks about St John's wort. A *Cochrane Review* suggests that evidence regarding efficacy of St John's wort is inconsistent and confusing. Hence if depression needs treatment, prescription drugs are recommended.

SF agrees to take amitriptyline, which is prescribed in the therapeutic dose for depression. She is advised about the potential side-effects and how to deal with them (Box 13.4). SF is aware that antidepressant medications must be taken regularly for 3–4 weeks (in some cases up to eight weeks) before full therapeutic effect occurs. Since SF's negative attitude may be contributing to her depression, she is also offered cognitive behavioural therapy (CBT).

Box 13.3 Suicide risk factors

Psychosocial and clinical
Hopelessness
Caucasian race
Male gender
Advanced age
Living alone

History
Prior suicide attempts
Family history of suicide attempts
Family history of substance abuse

Diagnostic
General medical illness
Psychosis
Substance abuse

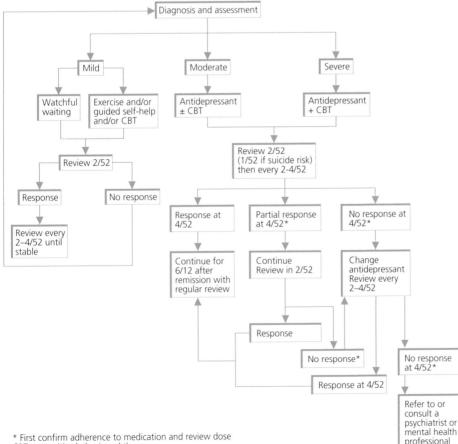

* First confirm adherence to medication and review dose
CBT = cognitive behavioural therapy

Figure 13.1 Overview of management of depression
Source: based on National Institute for Health and Clinical Excellence (NICE) CG23 Depression (amended). *Management of Depression in Primary and Secondary Care*. London: NICE, 2007. www.nice.org.uk/CG23.

Table 13.1 Side-effects profiles of commonly prescribed antidepressant medications

	Anticholinergic	Central nervous system			Cardiovascular		Gastrointestinal	
		Sedation	Headache	Agitation/ insomnia	Cardiac arrhythmia	Orthostatic	Nausea/GI symptoms	Weight gain (+) or loss (−)
Tricyclics								
amitriptyline	++++	+++++	0	0	+++	+++	0	++++
doxepin	+++	++++	0	0	++	++	0	+++
imipramine	+++	+++	0	0/+	+++	++++	+	+++
nortriptyline	++	++	0	0	++	+	0	+
SSRIs								
citalopram	0/+	0/+	transient	+	0	0	+++	0
fluoxetine	0	0	transient	++	0	0	+++	− −
paroxetine	+	0/+	transient	++	0	0	+++	0
sertraline	0	0/+	transient	++	0	0	+++	−
SNRI								
venlafaxine	+	+	transient	++	+	0	++	−
NaSSA								
mirtazepine	++	+++	0	0	0	+	0	++

SSRI = Selective serotonin reuptake inhibitor.
SNRI = Serotonin and noradrenaline reuptake inhibitor.
NaSSA = Noradrenergic and specific serotonergic antidepressant.

Table 13.2 Efficacy of antidepressants in the prevention of migraine

	Quality of evidence	Scientific effect	Clinical impression of effect
Tricyclics			
amitriptyline	A	+++	+++
doxepin	C	?	+
imipramine	C	?	+
nortriptyline	C	?	+++
SSRIs			
citalopram	?	?	+
fluoxetine	B	+	+
paroxetine	C	?	+
sertraline	C	?	+
SNRI			
venlafaxine	C	?	+
NaSSA			
mirtazepine	C	?	+

Quality of evidence
? No or insufficient data.
A. Multiple, well-designed randomized clinical trials, directly relevant to the recommendation, yielded a consistent pattern of findings.
B. Some evidence from randomized clinical trials supported the recommendation, but the scientific support was not optimal.
C. The US Headache Consortium achieved consensus on the recommendation in the absence of relevant randomized controlled trials.

Scientific effect measures
+ The effect of the medication is either not statistically or not clinically significant (i.e. less than the minimal clinically significant benefit).
++ The effect of the medication is statistically significant and exceeds the minimally clinically significant benefit.
+++ The effect is statistically significant and far exceeds the minimally clinically significant benefit.
? No or insufficient data.

Clinical impression of effect
+ Somewhat effective: few people get clinically significant improvement.
++ Effective: some people get clinically significant improvement.
+++ Very effective: most people get clinically significant improvement.

Source: adapted from US Headache Consortium. *Evidence-based Guidelines for Migraine Headache in the Primary Care Setting: Pharmacological Management for Prevention of Migraine.* www.americanheadachesociety.org/professionalresources/USHeadacheConsortiumGuidelines.asp

Box 13.4 **Antidepressant side-effects: advice to patients**

When you start antidepressants you may notice some unwanted side-effects before the benefits become apparent. These are usually mild and typically resolve within a few weeks of starting treatment, around the time that benefits kick in. The most common unwanted effects are listed below, together with some tips to help you deal with them. If you experience any severe or unusual reactions, you should always contact your doctor.

Tricyclic antidepressants (e.g. amitriptyline, doxepin, imipramine, nortriptyline, prothiadin)
- Dry mouth: sip water; chew sugarless gum; clean your teeth regularly.
- Constipation: increase your intake of water, fresh and dried fruits, vegetables and high-fibre cereals.
- Bladder symptoms: it is usual to find that you do not need to pass urine as often. Contact your doctor if it is difficult or painful to urinate.
- Sexual problems: this is a common problem with depression. Drugs can further reduce libido and make it more difficult to reach orgasm. Speak to your doctor.
- Blurred vision: this is most likely to occur early in treatment and usually resolves with time.
- Drowsiness: some antidepressants have a sedative effect. This can help poor sleep at night. If you feel drowsy or sedated during the day, you should not drive or operate heavy equipment. Taking a single evening dose a couple of hours before bedtime can minimise daytime drowsiness.

Selective serotonin reuptake inhibitors (SSRIs, e.g. citalopram, fluoxetine, paroxetine, sertraline)
- Headaches: daily headaches, even headaches similar to migraine, are common in the first few weeks of treatment but usually resolve in time.
- Nausea: this usually resolves with time.
- Nervousness and sleep disruption: these usually resolve with time, but discuss this with your doctor as you may need to consider reducing the dose or changing the time that you dose.
- Sexual problems: this is a common problem with depression. Drugs can further reduce libido and make it more difficult to reach orgasm. Speak to your doctor.

SF asks how this is going to help her headaches. If episodic tension-type headache is associated with depression, effective treatment of depression should resolve both conditions.

SF is reviewed two weeks later and reports that she is sleeping much better, but is very lethargic during the day. She has not noticed any improvement in mood or headache.

After a further two weeks, SF feels much the same and has noticed weight gain. She is not keen to increase the amitriptyline. She can now control the menstrual migraine. She is changed to an SSRI and advised about potential side-effects and how to manage them. Side-effects due to high levels of serotonin include headache, restlessness and gastrointestinal upset. In a study of 58 patients with migraine, headache was the most troublesome adverse event and was reported by 29% when starting sertaline and 43% following a dose increase. In the first 4 weeks after sertraline was started, the average number of migraine days was increased by 7.8% [95%CI 3.5–11.4] compared to baseline.

Several authorities have raised concern about the potential interaction between triptans and SSRIs and risk of serotonin syndrome. The symptoms of serotonin syndrome include euphoria, drowsiness, sustained rapid eye movement, overreaction of the reflexes, rapid muscle contraction and relaxation in the ankle causing abnormal movements of the foot, clumsiness, restlessness, feeling drunk and dizzy, muscle contraction and relaxation in the jaw, sweating, intoxication, muscle twitching, rigidity, high body temperature, shivering and diarrhoea. If the offending medication is discontinued, the condition will often resolve on its own within 24 hours. Reports of serotonin syndrome are rare and the combination of SSRIs and triptans is often recommended in clinical practice. However, all patients should be carefully monitored, as severe cases of serotonin syndrome can result in loss of consciousness and death.

At the next two-weekly review, SF reports that the SSRI is less sedating, although it initially made her feel sick and she had daily headaches. Four weeks later, the headaches are less frequent and her mood has improved. She thinks that the CBT is helping her confidence.

Referral

Moderate depression can usually be managed in primary care (Figure 13.2). Referral to mental healthcare professionals should be considered if there is no response to the change in treatment or if her mood deteriorates (Figure 13.1). If mood improves but headaches fail to respond to standard strategies, consider referral to a headache specialist.

Final diagnosis

1. Menstrually-related migraine without aura
2. Headache attributed to major depressive disorder (Box 13.5)

Management plan

SF is advised to continue the SSRI for at least six months after remission of depression. She continues with symptomatic treatment for menstrual migraine.

Outcome

SF continues the SSRI for seven months, after which she gradually reduces the dose over one month. She no longer has daily headaches and controls her menstrual attacks with symptomatic treatment only.

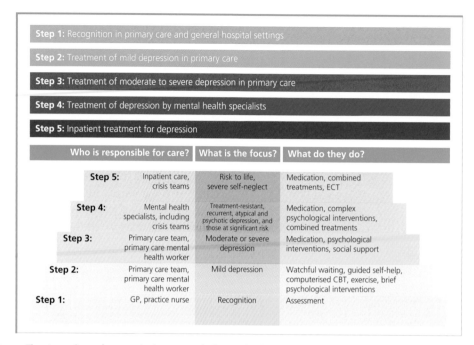

Figure 13.2 Stepped care. The stepped care framework aims to match the needs of people with depression to the most appropriate services, depending on the characteristics of their illness and their personal and social circumstances. Each step represents increased complexity of intervention, with higher steps assuming interventions in previous steps.

Source: National Institute for Health and Clinical Excellence (NICE) CG23 Depression (amended). *Management of Depression in Primary and Secondary Care.* London: NICE, 2007. www.nice.org.uk/CG23. Reproduced with permission.

Box 13.5 **International Classification of Headache Disorders. Diagnostic criteria for headache attributed to psychiatric disorder**

Headache attributed to major depressive disorder
Diagnostic criteria

A. Headache, no typical characteristics known, fulfilling criteria C–E
B. Presence of major depressive disorder fulfilling DSM-IV criteria:
  1. one or more episodes in which, during the same two-week period, at least five of the following symptoms are present:
    a) depressed mood
    b) markedly diminished interest or pleasure
    c) weight or appetite change
    d) insomnia or hypersomnia
    e) psychomotor agitation or retardation
    f) fatigue or loss of energy
    g) feeling of worthlessness or excessive or inappropriate guilt
    h) diminished ability to concentrate or indecisiveness
    i) recurrent thoughts of death, suicidal idea, plan or attempt
  2. occurring in the absence of any manic or hypomanic episodes
  3. not better accounted for by bereavement and not due to the direct physiological effects of a medical condition or substance
C. Headache occurs exclusively during major depressive episodes
D. Headache resolves or greatly improves within three months after the major depressive disorder is in full remission
E. Headache is not attributed to another cause

Source: Headache Classification Subcommittee of the International Headache Society (IHS). *The International Classification of Headache Disorders* (2nd edition). *Cephalalgia* 2004; **24** (suppl 1): 1–160.

Further reading

Frediani F, Villani V. Migraine and depression. *Neurol Sci* 2007; **28**:(suppl 2) S161–5.

Kroenke K, Spitzer RL, Williams JBW. The PHQ-9. Validity of a brief depression measure. *J Gen Intern Med* 2001; **16**: 606–13.

Linde K, Mulrow CD, Berner M, Egger M. St John's wort for depression. *Cochrane Database of Systematic Reviews* 2005, Issue 2. Art. No.: CD000448. DOI: 10.1002/14651858.CD000448.pub2

NICE. Clinical Guideline 23 (amended). *Depression: Management of Depression in Primary and Secondary Care.* London: NICE, 2007. www.nice.org.uk/CG23

Simon GE, VonKorff M, Piccinelli M, et al. An international study of the relation between somatic symptoms and depression. *N Eng J Med* 1999; **341**: 1329–35.

US Headache Consortium. *Evidence-based Guidelines for Migraine Headache In the Primary Care Setting: Pharmacological Management for Prevention of Migraine.* www.americanheadachesociety.org/professionalresources/USHeadacheConsortiumGuidelines.asp

CHAPTER 14

Pain in the Temple

R. Allan Purdy

OVERVIEW

- Headaches in the elderly always require investigation for a secondary causation
- The history is important as on examination there are few clinical signs
- Systemic symptoms have to be sought to make the diagnosis
- Failure to diagnose secondary causes has serious consequences

CASE HISTORY

The man with boring temporal headache

JS is a 72-year-old man with a three-month history of left temporal headache. The headache is moderately severe and boring in nature and without relieving or aggravating factors. Over time the headache is gradually worsening and he has begun to feel ill. On direct questioning he admits that when he eats he is developing pain in his jaw and now pain in his tongue. He has noticed increasing fatigue and some weight loss. In the past few weeks he has noticed recurrent episodes of transient loss of vision in his left eye, coming down like a curtain. On examination he looks 'sick' and in distress, and has one prominent physical finding.

History

Character questions

JS has a boring steady headache which is not specific for any primary or secondary headache disorder and one which could be a chronic daily headache since it is present more than 15 days a month and is longer than four hours in duration.

Cause questions

JS did not report any triggering or relieving factors. This is very important since most primary headaches, including migraine, tension-type headache and cluster headache, have definite modifying factors. As this is associated with a progressive worsening

over time, it is a definite 'red flag' with respect to looking for a secondary cause.

General symptoms

JS feels unwell and has fatigue and weight loss. These symptoms on their own could suggest a systemic disease or a malignant process, which can present with headaches as well. However, one should consider the differential diagnosis more broadly in any patient with constitutional symptoms. Also patients with primary headache can have anorexia (tension-type headache) and nausea and vomiting (migraine), but these symptoms are episodic. Further, at 72 JS's age starts to play a role in the diagnostic formulation.

Jaw and tongue pain

JS has volunteered these symptoms and they need to be evaluated carefully. They suggest some need for activity to bring them on and are termed jaw and tongue claudication respectively. They suggest that the blood supply to the muscles is compromised to ischaemic levels during eating and chewing, so that the subsequent pain is most likely ischaemic in nature.

Visual symptoms

The visual symptoms here are classic for amaurosis fugax, which implies reduced blood supply to the central retinal artery. The classic 'blind coming down' nature of the symptom is based on the anatomical blood supply to the retina; that is, the lower vessels become involved first, then the upper arterioles.

State of health otherwise

There are no other important features in his history. He has had some mild hypertension over time and gall bladder removal.

Examination

BP 140/90, regular pulse of 76. He looked ill, but had a normal general examination, except that he had tenderness on palpation of the extracranial vessels in his left temporal region; fundi showed some atherosclerotic and hypertensive arteriole changes, but these were not marked and his neurological examination was otherwise unremarkable.

Investigations

Preliminary blood work, including a complete blood count, C-reactive protein (CRP) and erythrocyte sedimentation rate (ESR),

ABC of Headache. Edited by A. MacGregor & A. Frith.
© 2009 Blackwell Publishing, ISBN 978-1-4051-7066-6.

were ordered, along with an ECG, chest x-ray and baseline unenhanced CT scan.

Diagnosis

Differential diagnosis

This appears to be a secondary headache in an older patient. One might think of a transient ischaemic attack (TIA) because of the visual symptoms and, if so, be concerned about carotid artery disease due to atherosclerosis. However, daily headache is unusual in a TIA. Further, the headache is progressive, so an alternative vascular diagnosis such as arteritis should be kept in mind, specifically temporal or giant cell arteritis. A less likely concern is cardiac emboli from non-bacterial endocarditis associated with an underlying malignancy, which might fit with some of the general and systemic symptoms.

Preliminary diagnosis

The visual symptoms are very characteristic of giant cell arteritis (Box 14.1). Jaw and tongue claudication, as well as pain in the shoulders (polymyalgia rheumatica), are also typical of the diagnosis (Box 14.2). Systemic symptoms of being and 'looking' ill are classic, but not specific. Temporal arteritis is a systemic disorder and is really a misnomer since other major arteries can be involved, including the carotid, basilar and coronary arteries, which could cause a major stroke or myocardial infarction. Hence the better term is giant cell arteritis. The headache in giant cell arteritis is not specific but is an early alert to the diagnosis in the case of any elderly patient (Boxes 14.3 and 14.4). The pain is usually located over the temporal artery region and is the commonest presenting symptom of the disorder.

It should be noted that an anterior ischaemic optic neuropathy (AION) can occur in patients with giant cell arteritis. AION can lead to permanent blindness if not recognized and treated. Treatment with corticosteroids can reduce the incidence of blindness to less than 25%. Nevertheless deterioration of vision has been reported in up to 17% of treated patients. Once visual loss occurs, it is usually severe and irreversible.

The diagnosis was supported by the clinical observation of a swollen, tortuous and painful left temporal artery (Figure 14.1).

Initial management

Initial management is shown in Box 14.5.

Blood tests

The results of the blood tests can be very informative and strongly support the diagnosis in this case. The full blood count (FBC) showed a microcytic anaemia, the ESR was 125, with a CRP of 42. JS's serum chemistry and ECG were essentially normal.

Treat with corticosteroids

Treatment here is mandatory and should be commenced as early as possible to prevent major complications of the arteritis, especially loss of vision, usually due to an AION. The treatment is oral steroids with the dosage range of prednisolone of 40–80 mg/day, although 60 mg/day or above has been more commonly suggested than lower doses (Box 14.6).

CT scan

A CT scan is reasonable in this case as JS could have a systemic malignancy with secondary brain metastases or small infarctions

---

Box 14.1 **Ocular manifestations of giant cell arteritis**

- Amaurosis fugax
- Diplopia
- Eye pain
- Visual hallucinations
- Visual loss

Box 14.2 **Systemic manifestations of giant cell arteritis**

- Headache
- Jaw claudication
- Tongue claudication
- Abnormal temporal arteries
- Polymyalgia rheumatica
- General malaise
- Fatigue
- Weight loss
- Depression
- Fever
- Night sweats

Box 14.3 **American College of Rheumatology 1990 criteria for the classification of giant cell (temporal) arteritis***

1. Age at disease onset >50 years: Development of symptoms or findings beginning at age 50 or older
2. New headache: New onset of or new type of localized pain in the head
3. Temporal artery abnormality: Temporal artery tenderness to palpation or decreased pulsation, unrelated to arteriosclerosis of cervical arteries
4. Elevated erythrocyte sedimentation rate: ESR >50 mm/h by the Westergren method
5. Abnormal artery biopsy: Biopsy specimen with artery showing vasculitis characterized by a predominance of mononuclear cell infiltration or granulomatous inflammation, usually with multinucleated giant cells

*For purposes of classification, a patient shall be said to have giant cell (temporal) arteritis if at least three of these five criteria are present. The presence of any three or more criteria yields a sensitivity of 93.5% and a specificity of 91.2%.
Source: Hunder GG, Bloch DA, Michel BA, Stevens MB, Arend WP, Calabrese LH, et al. The American College of Rheumatology 1990 criteria for the classification of giant cell arteritis. *Arthritis Rheum* 1990; **33**: 1122–8.

Box 14.4 **International Classification of Headache Disorders. Diagnostic criteria for headache attributed to giant cell arteritis**

Previously used terms: Temporal arteritis, Horton's disease
Diagnostic criteria:
A. Any new persisting headache fulfilling criteria C and D
B. At least one of the following:
    1. swollen tender scalp artery with elevated ESR and/or CRP
    2. temporal artery biopsy demonstrating giant cell arteritis
C. Headache develops in close temporal relation to other symptoms and signs of giant cell arteritis
D. Headache resolves or greatly improves within three days of high-dose steroid treatment

Comment: Of all arteritides and collagen vascular diseases, giant cell arteritis is the disease most conspicuously associated with headache due to inflammation of head arteries, mostly branches of the external carotid artery. The following points should be stressed:

• The variability in the characteristics of headache and other associated symptoms of giant cell arteritis (polymyalgia rheumatica, jaw claudication) are such that any recent persisting headache in a patient >60 years of age should suggest giant cell arteritis and lead to appropriate investigations
• Recent repeated attacks of amaurosis fugax associated with headache are very suggestive of giant cell arteritis and should prompt urgent investigations
• The major risk is blindness due to anterior ischaemic optic neuropathy. This can be prevented by immediate steroid treatment
• The interval between visual loss in one eye and in the other is usually less than one week
• Risks of cerebral ischaemic events and of dementia
• On histological examination, the temporal artery may appear uninvolved in some areas (skip lesions), pointing to the need for serial sectioning
• Duplex scanning of the temporal arteries may visualize the thickened arterial wall (as a halo on axial sections) and may help to select the site for biopsy

Source: Headache Classification Subcommittee of the International Headache Society (IHS). *The International Classification of Headache Disorders* (2nd edition). *Cephalalgia* 2004; **24** (suppl 1): 1–160.

Box 14.5 **Initial management of suspected giant cell arteritis**

• Obtain results of blood work
• Commence treatment with corticosteroids
• CT baseline scan to look for other diagnoses in this case
• Carotid duplex dopplers in this case to rule out carotid disease with TIA
• Temporal artery biopsy

Box 14.6 **A structured regime for treatment of giant cell arteritis with steroids**

1. No visual involvement:
    Prednisolone orally 60 mg daily for seven days, then 50 mg daily for seven days, then 40 mg daily for seven days then further gradual reduction in treatment according to symptoms and other markers of disease activity.
2. With visual involvement:
    Intravenous hydrocortisone 200 mg immediately and prednisolone orally 80 mg daily for three days followed by the above regimen.

Source: Ray-Chaudhuri N, Kine DA, Tijani SO, et al. Effect of prior steroid treatment on temporal artery biopsy findings in giant cell arteritis. *Br J Ophthalmol* 2002; **86(5)**: 530–2.

from prior carotid TIAs or cardiac microemboli. In his case this test was normal for age and that is the usual finding in this disorder.

Carotid Dopplers

Again this test is reasonable since JS presented with amaurosis, which usually is due to artery-to-artery embolism from the internal carotid artery to the ophthalmic artery and retinal vessels. However, in JS's case the test was normal.

Temporal artery biopsy

A temporal artery biopsy is an important test to do as soon as reasonable. A good section of artery is required to avoid skip lesions. It should be done by an experienced surgeon and read by a pathologist familiar with the disorder. Delay of therapy, however, is not warranted while waiting for the biopsy. If the biopsy is positive, treatment should continue. If the biopsy is negative or equivocal, treatment should be guided by clinical impressions and/or other laboratory tests, especially the ESR. Figure 14.2 shows typical arteritis as seen in this classic presentation of giant cell arteritis.

Referral

Patients with giant cell arteritis can be managed by most general practitioners, but referral to a neurologist, rheumatologist or general physician may be helpful for diagnosis and ongoing management. As indicated, surgery and pathology are involved early. An ophthalmological opinion can be most helpful for assessment and follow-up if eye symptoms are confusing or need reviewing.

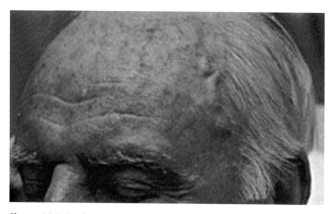

Figure 14.1 Swollen, tortuous temporal artery

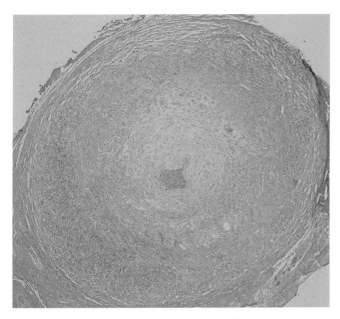

Figure 14.2 Temporal artery biopsy, with arteritis obliterating the lumen

Final diagnosis

Giant cell arteritis with visual symptoms, headache and systemic symptoms.

Management plan

The duration of therapy depends on JS's clinical course and follow-up assessments. Most patients require high-dose steroids for several weeks and this may last up to a year or longer. The addition of steroid-sparing or other immunosuppressive agents such as azathioprine or methotrexate are sometimes used. Long-term problems with steroids are to be avoided and managed. Patients have to be aware of these prior to starting therapy. Nevertheless, in this disorder the therapy clearly appears to outweigh the potential complications of the disease.

Outcome

After receiving prednisolone orally JS's symptoms started to subside within hours. The next day he was headache-free on 60 mg per day. He continued on this dose for a month and then it was gradually tapered and discontinued several months later as he became asymptomatic in all respects and his blood tests normalized.

Further reading

Caselli RJ, Hunder GG. Giant cell arteritis and polymyalgia rheumatica. In *Wolff's Headache and Other Head Pain*, 7th edition Eds Silberstein SD, Lipton RB, Dalessio DJ. Oxford: Oxford University Press, 2001: 525–35.

Goodwin, J. Temporal arteritis. *Medlink*. http://www.medlink.com.

Hunder GG, Bloch DA, Michel BA, et al. The American College of Rheumatology 1990 criteria for the classification of giant cell arteritis. *Arthritis Rheum* 1990; **33(8)**: 1122–8.

Loddenkemper T, Sharma P, Katzan I, Plant GT. Risk factors for early visual deterioration in temporal arteritis. *J Neurol Neurosurg Psychiatry* 2007; **78(11)**: 1255–9.

Rahman W, Rahman FZ. Giant cell (temporal) arteritis: an overview and update. *Surv Ophthalmol* 2005; **50(5)**: 415–28.

Ray-Chaudhuri N, Kine DA, Tijani SO, et al. Effect of prior steroid treatment on temporal artery biopsy findings in giant cell arteritis. *Br J Ophthalmol* 2002; **86(5)**: 530–2.

CHAPTER 15

Facial Pain

David W. Dodick

CASE HISTORY

The woman with pain in the jaw
BF is 52. She has had pain in the left side of the face for the past two months. The pain occurs daily and is characterized by sharp and extremely severe jolts of pain, each lasting about 1–2 seconds and occurring more than 50 times a day. The pain is located in the mid-portion of the face and along the jaw. The pain can occur spontaneously or may be triggered by touching the left side of the face, talking or chewing. After a series of jolts, there is a period of minutes during which the pain will disappear and cannot be triggered.

History

How many different headache types does the patient experience?

BF has only one type of pain. When she is not experiencing these severe lancinating jabs of pain, she is pain-free.

Time questions

The pain began two months ago. She has not had one day without the pain since it began. The pain recurs throughout the day, and is mainly related to activities. The more she talks or chews, the more severe the pain. Each stab of pain lasts only 1–2 seconds, but she

ABC of Headache. Edited by A. MacGregor & A. Frith.
© 2009 Blackwell Publishing, ISBN 978-1-4051-7066-6.

may experience a dozen or more stabs of pain in succession. There is a brief respite from the pain lasting minutes after each volley of stabs, during which time the pain cannot be triggered.

Character questions

The character of the pain is stabbing, piercing or jolt-like. The pain feels superficial. There is no associated paraesthesia or loss of sensation. When she experiences dozens of stabs in rapid succession there is a lingering pain in the same distribution as the stabbing pain, which persists for up to 30 minutes. She rates the pain on a 10-point severity scale as 10/10.

Cause questions

The pain began without injury, illness or provocation. However, the stabbing pain can be triggered by touching the face just below the left maxilla, or angle of the mouth on the left. The pain can also be triggered by talking, chewing and even a light breeze on the face.

Response to headache questions

BF feels agitated during these painful paroxysms. It is difficult for her to sit still, though she does not find any particular position comfortable. She has not found simple analgesics to be helpful. Oral opioid medications have similarly not been helpful and have only caused sedation and constipation. She was treated with two courses of antibiotics on the assumption that a sinus infection was causing the pain, but the pain has not resolved. She has not been able to work over the past two months. Because chewing triggers the pain, she has avoided eating and has lost more than 10 kg in weight.

State of health between attacks

In between attacks BF feels quite well. She is anxious, anticipating the next flurry of attacks. Her mood is poor because of the pain, inability to eat and inability to work or socialize.

Examination

Vital signs were within normal limits, and general physical and neurological examination was normal, except for dry mucous membranes, blunted affect and wincing with each paroxysm of pain. Pain in the distribution of the maxillary and mandibular branches of the trigeminal nerve (V2 and V3) could be triggered by light tactile stimulation of the left side of the face, just under the left maxilla. Facial sensation and corneal reflexes were intact, and there were no intra-oral lesions, tenderness over the frontal or maxillary sinuses, and no crepitus or pain to palpation over the temporomandibular joints.

Investigations

Complete blood count and serum chemistry were normal. Brain MRI with gadolinium was also normal. However, high resolution images through the posterior fossa revealed a small artery which contacted the left trigeminal nerve at the cisternal segment (Figure 15.1 a–c).

Diagnosis

Differential diagnosis

The differential diagnosis includes classical trigeminal neuralgia and symptomatic trigeminal neuralgia (Boxes 15.1 and 15.2). This patient has all the typical features of classical trigeminal neuralgia, including age and gender, V2 and V3 distribution, presence of trigger zones and typical triggers (chewing, talking), and the lack of persistent background interictal pain and paresthesias or sensory loss in the face. The pain of trigeminal neuralgia involves V2 or V3 or both in 95% of patients. Pain localized to V1 occurs in less than 5% of patients (Figure 15.2). A dull, aching discomfort may persist for up to 30 minutes, or even several hours, following an especially long or intense episode of pain.

Pain that spreads to involve the ear, occiput, neck or chest should cast doubt on the diagnosis. Bilateral pain is invariably associated with a secondary cause. In addition, suspicion of a secondary cause should arise when a continuous pain is punctuated by paroxysms of pain or when sensory loss in the trigeminal nerve distribution occurs. Trigeminal neuralgia in a patient under 40 years should also be investigated for a secondary cause such as multiple sclerosis or compressive lesions involving the trigeminal nerve. Even when the

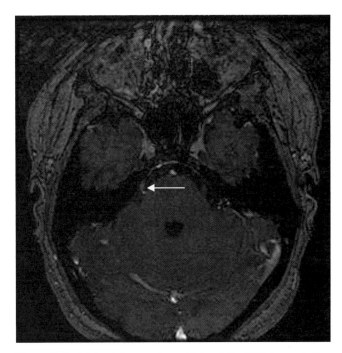

Figure 15.1b Axial gadolinium enhanced T-1 weighted MRI demonstrating vessel abutting trigeminal nerve

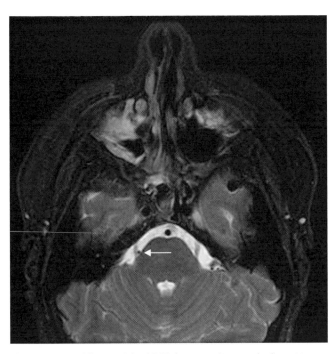

Figure 15.1a Axial T-2 weighted MRI demonstrating vessel adjacent to trigeminal nerve

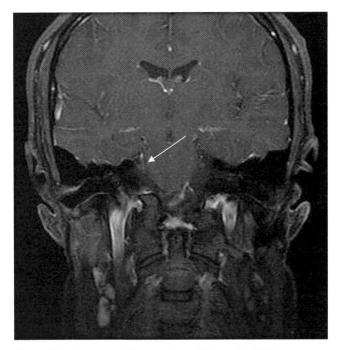

Figure 15.1c Coronal gadolinium enhanced T-1 weighted MRI demonstrating vessel coursing around nerve

Box 15.1 **International Classification of Headache Disorders. Diagnostic criteria for classical trigeminal neuralgia**

Trigeminal neuralgia is a unilateral disorder characterized by brief, electric shock-like pains, abrupt in onset and termination, limited to the distribution of one or more divisions of the trigeminal nerve. Pain is commonly evoked by trivial stimuli, including washing, shaving, smoking, talking and/or brushing the teeth (trigger factors) and frequently occurs spontaneously. Small areas in the nasolabial fold and/or chin may be particularly susceptible to the precipitation of pain (trigger areas). The pain usually remits for variable periods.

Diagnostic criteria
A. Paroxysmal attacks of pain lasting from a fraction of 1 second to 2 minutes, affecting one or more divisions of the trigeminal nerve and fulfilling criteria B and C
B. Pain has at least one of the following characteristics:
  1. intense, sharp, superficial or stabbing
  2. precipitated from trigger areas or by trigger factors
C. Attacks are stereotyped in the individual patient
D. There is no clinically evident neurological deficit
E. Not attributed to another disorder

Source: Headache Classification Subcommittee of the International Headache Society (IHS). *The International Classification of Headache Disorders* (2nd edition). *Cephalalgia* 2004; **24**(suppl 1): 1–160.

Box 15.2 **International Classification of Headache Disorders. Diagnostic criteria for symptomatic trigeminal neuralgia**

Pain indistinguishable from classic trigeminal neuralgia but caused by a demonstrable structural lesion other than vascular compression.

Diagnostic criteria
A. Paroxysmal attacks of pain lasting from a fraction of 1 second to 2 minutes, with or without persistence of aching between paroxysms, affecting one or more divisions of the trigeminal nerve and fulfilling criteria B and C
B. Pain has at least one of the following characteristics:
  1. intense, sharp, superficial or stabbing
  2. precipitated from trigger areas or by trigger factors
C. Attacks are stereotyped in the individual patient
D. A causative lesion, other than vascular compression, has been demonstrated by special investigations and/or posterior fossa exploration

Source: Headache Classification Subcommittee of the International Headache Society (IHS). *The International Classification of Headache Disorders* (2nd edition). *Cephalalgia* 2004; **24**(suppl 1): 1–160.

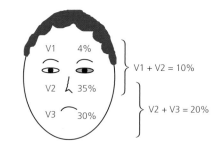

Figure 15.2 Distribution of trigeminal neuralgia

Box 15.3 **Clinical features of neuralgic pain**

- Paroxysmal and brief (2–10 seconds)
- Sudden, intense, stabbing
- Precipitated by certain activities (brushing, chewing, swallowing)
- Associated with trigger zones
- Pain-free intervals between paroxysms of pain
- No demonstrable cranial nerve lesion or abnormal physical sign

Box 15.4 **Diagnostic evaluation of non-neuralgic pain**

- Baseline haematological and chemistry studies, sedimentation rate
- MRI with gadolinium evaluating brain, posterior fossa, jaw, neck (soft tissues, bone, nasopharynx, sphenoid sinus)
- Otolaryngology, dental, and ophthalmology consultation
- Chest x-ray or chest CT if index of suspicion high for malignancy

Three-dimensional gadolinium-enhanced MR angiography of the posterior fossa may show vascular compression in up to 90% of classic cases. When present, vascular compression may direct therapy since microvascular decompression surgery is considered to be more effective in these patients. Although impaired sensation and subjective feelings of facial numbness are usually absent in patients with classic trigeminal neuralgia, they may be present in 15–25% of patients. Patients with subjective or objective sensory loss are more likely to demonstrate vascular compression or extrinsic mass compression of the nerve on MRI.

In patients whose pain is not typically neuralgic, a thorough evaluation is necessary (Box 15.4). This is designed to exclude disease involving the pulmonary apex, nasopharynx, teeth, oral cavity and temporomandibular joint which may refer pain to the face.

Initial management

Medical therapy

Both medical and surgical therapy may be considered for patients with trigeminal neuralgia. Up to 50% of patients may experience remission for more than six months and approximately a third may experience only a single bout of pain. Therefore, medical therapy is appropriate in most patients as initial therapy. After approximately eight weeks of successful therapy with complete remission of pain, a slow drug taper over a similar period may be warranted.

features appear typical, studies with large numbers of patients suggest that up to 10% of patients with trigeminal neuralgia may harbour an intracranial lesion. This underscores the need to consider an MRI on every patient with trigeminal neuralgia, even in those who respond to medication and whose examination is normal.

Preliminary diagnosis

Classic trigeminal neuralgia is the most likely diagnosis. The clinical features are typical of neuralgic pain (Box 15.3).

Table 15.1 Medical treatments for trigeminal neuralgia

Drug	Initial daily dose	Maintenance daily dose
Carbamazepine	100 mg bd	200–1200 mg in 2–4 divided doses
Oxcarbazepine	150–300 mg bd	300–600 mg bd
Gabapentin	100 mg tds	300–600 mg tds
Lamotrigine	25 mg od	200–400 mg as a single dose or two divided doses
Baclofen	5–10 mg bd	30–60 mg in 2–4 divided doses
Clonazepam	0.5–1.0 mg tds	1.5–8 mg tds
Phenytoin	200 mg od	300–600 mg as a single dose or two divided doses
Pimozide	2 mg bd	4–12 mg bd
Valproic acid	250 mg bd	500–2000 mg in two divided doses

Recommended treatments are listed in Table 15.1. Before starting any of these medications, it is prudent to obtain a baseline complete blood count and serum chemistry as some of the recommended treatments may cause haematopoietic or systemic toxicity. As a general rule, all medications should be started at low dosages and titrated slowly according to the desired effect and side-effect profile. In this way, the lowest effective dose is achieved and the side-effects minimized. Monotherapy is a treatment goal, but in some patients combination therapy with two drugs used in smaller dosages may be more effective and better tolerated.

Carbamazepine and oxcarbazepine are often the first-line drugs for trigeminal neuralgia. As oxcarbazepine is not associated with bone marrow suppression, it is usually preferred. Hyponatremia may be seen in up to 5% of patients treated with either drug, so periodic monitoring of electrolyte concentrations is necessary in patients on long-term therapy.

Surgical therapy

Approximately 30% of patients will fail medical therapy and may require a surgical or ablative procedure. For elderly patients who are medically unfit for a more invasive surgical procedure, or in patients who require immediate relief, extracranial peripheral nerve denervation may be considered. Peripheral denervation is performed at the supraorbital notch for first-division pain, infra-orbital notch for maxillary-division pain, and the mental foramen for mandibular-division pain. Lidocaine and bupivicaine are used for temporary denervation, while more permanent denervation is achieved with alcohol, freezing and heating. Cutting or avulsing the nerve via neurectomy is also a surgical treatment option.

Percutaneous radiofrequency, glycerol or balloon compression trigeminal rhizotomy are the ablative procedures of choice. Each procedure has similar long-term success rates (60–85%) with acceptable operative morbidity. Facial sensory loss may occur with both procedures. Corneal anaesthesia, anaesthesia dolorosa, facial dysaesthesias and masseter muscle weakness are uncommon adverse events.

Gamma knife stereotactic radiosurgery, a procedure that delivers cobalt radiation to the cisternal segment of the trigeminal nerve at the root entry zone, has recently been approved by the UK's National Institute for Health and Clinical Excellence for treatment of trigeminal neuralgia, but access to this treatment is limited. The advantage of this procedure is its non-invasiveness, lack of general anaesthesia, favourable morbidity and absent mortality. The disadvantages include the 1–2-month delay between treatment and therapeutic effect and, similar to other ablative procedures, the small risk of facial sensory loss, dysaesthesias and recurrence of trigeminal neuralgia in up to a third of patients.

Microvascular decompression (MVD) is considered to be the definitive procedure for classic trigeminal neuralgia but it is often reserved for intractable cases because of the need for a craniotomy. It may also be considered in patients with V1 distribution pain because of the risk for corneal anaesthesia after ablative procedures and in young, medically refractory or recurrent post-surgical patients. At 10 years after MVD, 70% of patients continue to show excellent results. The procedure involves an occipital craniotomy and separation of the trigeminal nerve from a juxtaposed or adherent vessel using a synthetic material.

Referral

Specialist referral should be considered for the patient who does not respond to conventional treatment with first-line medications, for patients who desire surgical treatment or for patients who have contraindications to first-line medications.

Final diagnosis

Classic trigeminal neuralgia.

Outcome

BF started on oxcarbazepine at a dosage of 300 mg bd, which was increased to 600 mg bd after one week. Within two days, the patient's pain had lessened considerably. Improvement continued to accrue and 10 days after therapy began the patient was pain-free. Two months later, the patient continued to be pain-free. A slow taper was begun, reducing the dosage by 300 mg per week. The pain has not recurred.

Further reading

Anderson VC, Berryhill PC, Sandquist MA, Ciaverella DP, Nesbit GM, Burchiel KJ. High-resolution three-dimensional magnetic resonance angiography and three-dimensional spoiled gradient-recalled imaging in the evaluation of neurovascular compression in patients with trigeminal neuralgia: a double-blind pilot study. *Neurosurgery* 2006; **58(4)**: 666–73.

Bennetto L, Patel NK, Fuller G. Trigeminal neuralgia and its management. *BMJ* 2007; **334(7586)**: 201–5.

Hentschel K, Capobianco DJ, Dodick DW. Facial pain. *Neurologist* 2005; **11(4)**: 244–9.

Lopez BC, Hamlyn PJ and Zakrzewska JM. Systematic review of ablative neurosurgical techniques for the treatment of trigeminal neuralgia. *Neurosurgery* 2004; **54(4)**: 973–83.

Further resources

Specialist clinics

The City of London Migraine Clinic
22 Charterhouse Square
London EC1M 6DX
Tel: 020 7251 3322
Fax: 020 7490 2183
www.migraineclinic.org.uk

Professional organisations

British Association for the Study of Headache
c/o Dr Fayyaz Ahmed
Department of Neurology
Hull Royal Infirmary
Analby Road
Hull HU3 2JZ
www.bash.org.uk

International Headache Society
c/o Griffin Stone Moscrop & Co
41 Welbeck Street
London W1G 8EA
Email: carol.taylor@i-h-s.org
www.i-h-s.org

National Association for Premenstrual Syndrome
41 Old Road
East Peckham
Kent TN12 5AP
Tel: 0870 7772178
Helpline: 0870 7772177
www.pms.org.uk

Royal College of Psychiatrists
17 Belgrave Square
London SW1X 8PG
www.rcpsych.ac.uk
Select 'depression' on the drop down choice of topics on the home page for readable and well-researched booklets for the public available in a number of languages.

Lay organisations

Brain and Spine Foundation
Free Post LON10492
London SW9 6BR
Tel: 020 7793 5900
Helpline: 0808 808 1000
www.brainandspine.org.uk

Depression Alliance
212 Spitfire Studios
63–71 Collier Street
London N1 9BE
Tel: 0845 123 23 20
www.depressionalliance.org

Migraine Action Association
27 East Street
Leicester
Leicestershire LE1 6NB
Tel: 0116 275 8317
Fax: 0116 254 2023
www.migraine.org.uk

The Migraine Trust
2nd Floor
55–56 Russell Square
London WC1B 4HP
Tel: 020 7436 1336
Helpline: 020 7462 6601
Fax: 020 7436 2880
www.migrainetrust.org

Ouch (UK): The Organisation for the Understanding of
  Cluster Headache
74 Abbotsbury Road
Broadstone
Dorset BH8 9DD
Helpline: 01646 651 979
www.ouchuk.org

Samaritans
PO Box 9090
Stirling FK8 2SA
Helpline: 08457 90 90 90
Helpline (Ireland): 1850 60 90 90
Email: jo@samaritans.org
www.samaritans.org

Trigeminal Neuralgia Association (TNA UK)
PO Box 234
Oxted
Surrey RH8 8BE
Tel: 01883 370214
Email: help@tna.org.uk
www.tna.org.uk

World Headache Alliance
c/o Griffin Stone Moscrop & Co
41 Welbeck Street
London W1G 8EA
Email: info@w-h-a.org
www.w-h-a.org

Index